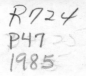

DOCTORS' DILEMMAS

Medical Ethics and Contemporary Science

Melanie Phillips
John Dawson

METHUEN, INC.
NEW YORK

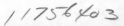

First published in 1985 in the United States of America
by Methuen, Inc. 733 Third Avenue, New York, N.Y. 10017

Library of Congress Cataloging in Publication Data

Phillips, Melanie, 1951—
  Doctors' Dilemmas.
  Bibliography p.
  1. Medical ethics. 2. Social medicine. 3. Medicine—
political aspects.
I. Dawson, John, 1946
II. Title.
R724   D3825   1985   174'.2   85-3039

ISBN 0-416-01111-X
ISBN 0-416-01121-7 Pbk

CONTENTS

PREFACE

When a doctor and a journalist get together to write a book, eyebrows may be raised. When the subject of the book is medical ethics, one of the most difficult and sensitive areas of medicine, the eyebrows may well disappear into the hairline completely. For one of the most controversial aspects of the medical ethics debate is the question of who is qualified to discuss it. For many doctors, the answer is clear. The ethical dimension to their work is so intimately related to their clinical judgement, and that judgement is itself so jealously guarded, that they are in no doubt at all that the only people qualified to pass any judgements about medical ethics are doctors themselves. To enlist the aid of a journalist to grapple with this most delicate of subjects would seem to many doctors incomprehensible to the point of treachery. Conversely, voices from outside the medical profession have recently begun to protest that the doctors have had it all their own way for far too long and that it is high time a variety of disciplines—law, philosophy, religion, and so on—were brought to bear on the problems of medical ethics. To such critics, collaboration with a doctor might well be viewed as a threat to a wholly dispassionate study, an automatic watering-down of the spirit of independent inquiry and debate.

We feel, however, that this kind of dissonance between doctors and medical laymen is unfortunate and an obstacle in the way of rational and well-informed discussion. It has not characterised the way we ourselves have worked in the past. The convergence of two perspectives, we felt, helped advance discussion and scrutiny of some of the most intractable problems arising in our complicated society, even though our particular contribution was modest. The purpose of writing this book is to explore in greater detail some of the underlying issues behind individual ethical problems that arise from time to time, issues that need to be considered away from the highly charged atmosphere of controversy characterising medical ethical dilemmas that arise from day to day. A crisis is a time to carry out a determined policy rather than to indulge in original thought and there seems to us to be good sense in exploring some parts of the boundary limiting the application of medical science before crises develop.

We feel strongly that such a public debate needs to take place. It has become a commonplace that advances in medicine have far outstripped our moral codes. Scientific achievements often score a kind of pyrrhic victory over suffering, in that they may create painful dilemmas where none previously existed. The baby who is born with multiple handicaps, for example, would only a short time ago have died at birth, yet now can be saved for what is potentially a life of suffering. At the other end of life, the old person suffering from senile dementia and a stroke might have been able to drift into an easeful death as a result of contracting pneumonia; now, we are able to counter that pneumonia and so prolong that life or, as some would see it, that dying process. We can now transplant hearts and other organs, so saving some patients from an otherwise certain early death; yet, because there is not enough money (or organs) to go round, someone has to decide who should be saved and who should be allowed to die. In other areas of experimentation, such as genetic engineering or *in vitro* fertilisation, we are able to interfere with nature to such a degree that the traditional aims of medicine are in danger of being subverted.

These dilemmas often revolve around some common ethical issues. For example, at the heart of the arguments over abortion, euthanasia, post-coital birth control and decisions about ending treatment lie the issues of where life actually begins and ends, and the often contradictory aims of observing the sanctity of life and enhancing its quality. Behind the specific debate over data protection and confidentiality, over the role of police surgeons or prison medical officers, lies the issue of the conflicting duties of a doctor towards his patient on the one hand and society at large on the other. Behind the immediate difficulties of doctors having to decide which of their kidney patients are to live or die lies the issue of rationing resources in a National Health Service that can never meet all the demands being made of it—and behind that in turn lies the potential conflict between the doctor's duties towards his patients and towards society.

We think that these issues should be argued in a reasoned, reasonable manner that ordinary people can understand so that they too can participate in the determination of a framework which can guide the application of medical science. Our book is aimed at the interested public, and is not written in medical, sociological or any other kind of jargon. We do not seek to preach; indeed, there will be some who will object that on many issues we have refrained from saying what we think is right or wrong. Our aim is to think through some of these difficult issues in order to expose arguments which might otherwise remain buried, to bring to light the many inconsistencies which have arisen as a result of a dearth of public discussion, to provide some idea of the scale of the problems we may be up against.

We are responsible for the opinions expressed in this book and the conclusions drawn from particular lines of argument. Nevertheless, we acknowledge with pleasure the help and advice we have received from the following people: Sir Douglas Black, Sir George Godber, Sir Norman Lindop, Mr Paul Sieghart, and Dr Michael Thomas.

Criticising draft chapters of someone else's book is no easy business. All of our critics are heavily occupied with other matters and their cheerful acceptance of an additional task, coupled with their careful, incisive criticism have made the latter stages of writing this book much easier than might have been the case. We are very grateful to each of them.

We have been helped greatly by Miss Valerie Booth and Miss Kate Saggers from the BMA's Press Department with research.

1
A FRAMEWORK FOR THE APPLICATION OF MEDICAL SCIENCE

Suddenly, medical ethics are fashionable. Articles and books on the subject are burgeoning, particularly in North America. In this country, a handful of court cases involving such topics as handicapped babies, euthanasia, teenage pregnancy and contraception has woken everyone up to the dilemmas that doctors face daily. A committee of inquiry set up by the government to grapple with the moral problems of *in vitro* fertilisation was a tacit admission of the possibility that advances in medical science might not be an entirely good thing.

Do we need medical ethics?

Doctors often say that the only ethics that matter to them are those that arise from day to day in their treatment of individual patients. Each case is different from the next; each demands what are often harsh choices, made under stress. The pressures of such a professional routine mean that many doctors become extremely impatient with ethical theories and even more impatient at the suggestion that they should be bound by them. Taken to its extreme, this would mean sanctioning a kind of moral anarchy in medicine. Those doctors who stress the importance of their on-the-job perspective, however, would also claim that they are bound by ancient ethical traditions. In many areas those traditions have been overtaken by advances in medical science and the complexities of modern society. It is a premise for this book that a code of medical ethics is necessary as a framework within which medical science can be applied. We believe that doctors must strike a bargain with the society they serve.

1

Doctors practise by using skills and knowledge which the
rest of us do not possess and which they use to heal sickness
and prolong life. They exercise great power over people who
are ill and vulnerable. Patients come to them in a dependent
position, not as equals. The potential for abuse of that
vulnerability is thus built into the relationship. In order to
safeguard the interests of those patients, doctors are obliged
to conform to an accepted code of behaviour because the
public is entitled to expect doctors to behave in certain ways.
If no ethical codes prevailed, doctors would behave unpre-
dictably and might not always act for the best. Robert
Veatch, in arguing against *ad hoc* decision-making in medicine, quoted Aristotle's dictum on whether it is better to be
governed by law or by the judgements of good individuals:
'A feast to which all guests contribute is better than a banquet
furnished by a single man.'

Medical science

Phenomenal advances have occurred in medical knowledge
and scientific skills, particularly in the years since the Second
World War. The power of medicine to prevent nature from
taking her course has been massively extended, and with that
greater power has come an almost intolerable extension of
moral choice. In many situations, doctors may now find it
difficult to know what to do for the best, whereas forty years
ago they simply would not have encountered similar
problems. When a patient suffered a heart attack, for
example, or a haemorrhage into the brain he or she would
quite likely have died. As soon as it became possible,
however, to keep the patient alive by artificial respiration, the
restoration of the normal balance of the body's chemistry,
and other improved resuscitation techniques, doctors were
faced with the dilemmas posed by their new ability. Was it
right to preserve life if the quality of that life was judged to be
poor? Should doctors make any decisions about the quality of
life, or should they preserve it at all costs? Was switching off
the life-support machine tantamount to murder? Even if it
wasn't, would it be seen as such by the relatives?

Or take the advances that have occurred in children's medicine—paediatrics. Once, severely handicapped babies would have died at birth or shortly after. When that happened, the doctor had no moral problem. Once he became able to extend those handicapped babies' lives, his problems started. Should he preserve all newborn life, however grave the handicap? If not, how should he judge where to draw the line? Whose interests should he take into account—the baby's, the parents' or society's? Was there a moral difference between killing a baby and letting it die? And so on. Or take the advances in drugs. New drugs are being developed all the time which have vastly extended the power of medicine to heal. But they have brought in their train new problems as well—iatrogenic illness, for example, where the patient actually becomes ill as a result of the treatment that is supposed to be a cure; or the dilemma of selecting patients to try out such new drugs, with the possible risk of harm to them. And so on.

Along with these increases in the power of scientific medicine, the horizons of medical practice have substantially changed. As Professor Basil Mitchell of Oriel College, Oxford, put it:

The scope of medical practice has been much enlarged and its aims therefore are less simply stated. It used to be the sole aim of medicine to cure disease, and physical disease at that. Hence the aim was the patient's health; and physical health was not hard to recognise, though it might be hard to define. But medical techniques may now be called upon for purposes which are not directly related to the health of the individual patient, e.g. in relation to contraception, abortion, sterilisation, sex changes and cosmetic operations of various kinds. Even insofar as the doctor's aim is still restoration to health, there are problems as to what constitutes health and, when not all the attributes of health are obtainable, which to prefer.

As a result of this widening of the doctor's role into the social field, the traditional ethical approach of the profession has come under increasing challenge. Professor Mitchell went on:

So long as the sole aim of medicine was the curing of disease, the doctor could claim without fear of contradiction that the entire field of medicine was subject to the ethics of his profession. Now there is a tendency on the part of many people to treat the doctor simply as a technician whose job it is to give the public what it wants. No doubt the conscience of the individual doctor has to be safeguarded, but the [collective] ethic of the medical profession as such is judged irrelevant. It is for society or the individual patient (who sees himself rather as a client or consumer than as a patient) to determine whether a man should be sterilised, or a foetus aborted, or a child of 12 placed on the pill. To the extent that this attitude is accepted, medical ethics are no longer coextensive with medical practice.

To a certain extent, Professor Mitchell seems to overstate the case. By no means everyone has thrown off the assumptions of the past; many people still very much regard themselves as patients and even want doctors to tell them what to do in situations where the doctor has no wish to do so. But by and large he has put his finger on the problem. Society has become more opinionated and challenging in this area, and thus there is a collision between the traditional, insular, professional approach and the collective wish of the community to tell doctors what is right and wrong. The change is not just confined to medicine and health; society's old obeisance to the doctrine of paternalism has been replaced by a far greater emphasis on autonomy and individual rights. People are becoming increasingly reluctant to accept in blind trust everything that the doctor tells them; they want a dialogue in which their own views are taken into account. But the trouble is that no one view prevails. There is no moral consensus, rather a moral pluralism. On matters of life and death or sexual morality, for example, a clamour of opposing opinions arises from the different camps of religious groups and secular humanists, within which there are still more divisions and dichotomies.

The medical profession still has a long way to go to meet the community in an adequate dialogue. But it should be recognised how far and how fast it has moved in a relatively short space of time. It hardly needs saying that modern medicine and the society it serves are far removed from the provisions of the Hippocratic Oath of the 4th century BC. But one does not have to travel back to ancient Greece to realise how the assumptions behind doctoring have changed. One has only to go back to 1970 and the British Medical Association's handbook, *Medical Ethics*, published that year. In retrospect, some of it makes remarkable reading. For example, under the heading 'Individual Responsiblity', the book states:

Formulation of rules is one thing, observance of them in the rough and tumble of professional practice is quite another. A measure of the integrity of the medical profession is to be found in the degree to which each practitioner recognises his personal responsibility for the preservation, through his own example, of the honour and dignity of the profession and the fact that serious breaches of its ethical code are relatively rare. The values of mutual goodwill and tolerance in the brotherhood of medicine cannot be over-emphasised.

It then goes on to quote a former chairman of the BMA's Central Ethical Committee:

In the relation of the practitioner to his fellows, while certain established customs and even rules are written and must be written, the principal influence to be cultivated is that of good fellowship. Most men know what is meant by 'cricket' and the spirit of the game. Difficulties and differences will arise, but most of them can be successfully met by mutual goodwill and recognition of the other person's point of view.

Such paternalistic, insular complacency would be unthinkable nowadays. Patients simply wouldn't stand for it; and the complexities of the moral dilemmas facing doctors today cannot be resolved by an assumption that the other chap is a decent sort. The simple cultural assumptions underlying the statement are insufficient for today's problems.

Existing ethical codes

A visitor from another planet might wonder, however, why ethical decision-making in medicine is suddenly so difficult.

After all, such an observer might point out, there is a positive plethora of codes of practice. Apart from the Hippocratic Oath itself, there is the Declaration of Geneva (1947) which is the modern restatement of the Hippocratic Oath, the Declaration of Helsinki on human experimentation, the Declaration of Oslo on therapeutic abortion, the Declaration of Tokyo on torture and degrading treatment, the Declaration of Sydney on death; not to mention various codes of medical ethics adopted by different countries and divers resolutions adopted by the World Medical Association (see Appendix). And indeed the codes do provide guidance on specific issues. But in many respects they have simply been outstripped by developments in society and in science. Society has changed and factors such as the autonomy of the individual, the need to tell the truth, the importance of distributive justice have become more important. These new principles conflict with the principles in the codes. The codes themselves contain conflicting principles, as we show in succeeding chapters; or they are too vague, and do not commit doctors to principles which many assume nevertheless to be the guiding principles of society. The codes do not recognise overtly the conflict between the claims of the individual against the requirements of society.

One of the gravest problems concerns the fundamental principle behind the Hippocratic Oath and the Declaration of Geneva—the commitment to patient-centred ethics, in which the physician is enjoined to produce benefit for the patient and to do the patient no harm. While no one would quarrel with these principles as stated, the problem arises in defining or assessing benefit or harm. When a doctor decides not to operate on a spina bifida baby to save its life, he does so because he is deciding that this is in the best interests of that child and its family. But in doing so, he is making highly contentious judgements about the likely quality of the child's life. If he doesn't operate and the child dies, how can the doctor be said to have acted in the child's best interests? How does the conclusion that such a child is better off dead square with the doctor's duty to remember his obligation to preserve life? How can he make the decision at all on the child's behalf, when, as some spina bifida sufferers have testified, it is possible to live fruitful and worthwhile lives even with such a handicap? But if the doctor does operate and saves the child's life, how can he square the likely suffering that the child will endure with the cardinal principle of medicine, *primum non nocere*—above all, do no harm?

In other words, if the doctor is enjoined to relieve pain and suffering, how can he actually prolong distress? These questions arise from the increasing sophistication of medical techniques and the relative simplicities of the various codes provide few answers.

Then there are the myriad contradictions. The Oath and the Declaration of Geneva stress the doctor's responsibility for the individual patient. But what about the best interests of all patients, society at large? What happens when the two interests come into conflict? Human experimentation is one example of this dilemma, where the interests of the individual may conflict with those of society. The Declaration of Helsinki provides guidelines to try to arrive at a balance of those interests, but the very fact that such a balance is thought necessary at all appears to conflict with the principles of the Declaration of Geneva: 'The health of my patient will be my first consideration. . . . Any act or advice which could weaken physical or mental resistance of a human being may be used only in his interest.' Or consider the vagueness in the codes, particularly about the sanctity of human life. It is widely believed among the lay public that doctors are required to save and preserve life at all costs. This is not true. The Hippocratic Oath makes no mention of it. The Declaration of Geneva fudges it: 'I will maintain the utmost respect for human life from the time of conception. . . . A doctor must always bear in mind the obligation of preserving human life.' Maintaining respect nevertheless allows doctors to carry out abortion or to fail to intervene to save a life that is considered damaged beyond value. Or does it? The point is that the codes tend to fall apart at the seams as soon as they are put under pressure, as we show in the course of this book. In addition, there are a number of principles that the codes do not begin to grapple with but which are important in our society. At the end of this book, we try to bring together some of the principles which appear to run through good decision-making in medicine in an attempt to provide some tools for the solution of moral dilemmas. That is different from the specific answers and directives of the Codes in the Appendix.

The conflict of principles

There is an underlying conflict that links all medical dilemmas. Crudely put, it is the conflict between absolute principles, which say that something is inherently right or wrong, and utilitarian principles, which stress the consequences of an action. (We are, of course, using these terms in a lay sense; they do not necessarily correspond to the definitions philosophers would use, and indeed in philosophy there are many variants of utilitarianism.) In other words, absolutists would say that some things are wrong and nothing can make them right. Utilitarians, on the other hand, would say that we must judge what to do for the best in a given situation. The difference was summed up by Professor Hare in this way:

For example, absolutists will say that because killing innocent people is always wrong, if you are in a situation in which if you do not kill one innocent person twenty other innocent people will die (though not by your hand) then you ought to be prepared to let the twenty die rather than become guilty of the death of one. But utilitarians will say that you have to act for the best in the circumstances, and save the twenty at the expense of one.

One of the clearest medical examples of this conflict is abortion. Leaving aside for a moment the crucial problem that people disagree over where life begins and over the value to be placed on the foetus, the conflict here is between those who say that destroying the foetus is inherently wrong and can never be right, and those who say that the question of whether it is right or wrong depends on the best results for society at large—the maximising of benefits. Or take the issue of confidentiality. The absolutist would say that medical confidentiality is sacrosanct and must never be broken. The utilitarian would say that it would depend on the circumstances, and in some cases the interests of society might best be served by a breach of the confidentiality rule. If these positions were adopted universally in their most extreme form, society would be a pretty unpleasant place in which to live. Take the question of the sanctity of life, for example. If the absolutist view prevailed, the highly scientific medicine that is practised now would try to save every single life from extinction regardless of the intolerable cost or consequences to other patients. Conversely, if the utilitarian view prevailed we might see many handicapped people subjected to euthanasia on the grounds that society's best interests were served by their removal. Our society is based upon an uneasy truce between the two points of view. But fresh medical dilemmas are created all the time by the conflict between the two positions.

There is, however, an attractive compromise that can be reached between the two viewpoints. It is sometimes called 'rule utility'. It allows the absolutists the inherent value of their arguments, but then measures that value against what is best for society at large. For example, take the question of euthanasia. The argument may go that one reason why it is wrong to take life in such circumstances is that once one has breached the principle of the sanctity of life one is on a dangerous 'slippery slope' in which people may be killed for a range of tendentious reasons. In other words, there are powerful utilitarian arguments to demonstrate that the absolutist principle is the right one to apply. Such a convergence could be used more generally. As Professor Veatch has argued:

Perhaps these right-making characteristics of actions are not independent principles but merely principles summarising a set of rules which, if followed, will produce the greatest good on balance. . . . This scheme is what philosophers have come to call the normative position of 'rule utility'. It probably comes very close to being able to account for our moral intuitions. It can usually explain, for example, why people ought to act justly, tell the truth, keep promises and respect freedom. Following such principles and the rules derived from them will tend to produce more benefit than following other principles and rules, even if in some individual cases more harm than good might be done.

Unfortunately, however, this does not solve the fundamental problem of medical ethics. It might provide us with some kind of rudimentary working structure to solve the problem of whether we should be an absolutist or a utilitarian society. But what it does not do is tell us how to rank those absolute principles in order to get the most beneficial result. For the principles still conflict. Doing good to the patient, for example, might conflict with the patient's autonomy. The patient might think that the doctor's idea of what is for the best is wrong, and a society which respects that autonomy then is faced with a conflict of principles. We have already touched on some of these conflicting theories, but it might be helpful to attempt a summary of the characteristics of the most important ones.

Principles

Doing good and not doing harm
Perhaps more than any other principles, these are deeply embedded in most people's assumptions about the codes that guide doctors. They are at the heart of the Hippocratic Oath: 'I will follow that system of regimen which, according to my ability and judgement, I consider for the benefit of my patients, and abstain from whatever is deleterious and mischievous.' The principle of 'above all, do no harm', however, is not always easy to put into practice. In some situations, doctors may be faced with a choice of harms. Catholic theology has come up with a justification for performing an action which may lead to an evil—the doctrine of double effect. Broadly speaking, this means doing something which in itself is either good or at most morally neutral, and which is intended to do good, but which may lead to something which is bad. The doctrine is mainly used in cases of dying patients, where for example the doctor may give pain-killing drugs which have the known side-effect of shortening life. According to the doctrine, provided the doctor is administering those drugs to relieve suffering and not to cause death, he is morally in the clear.

The prohibition against intentional harm, however, becomes more difficult in other cases—for example, the patient who (like Karen Quinlan in the United States) is in a permanent, comatose, vegetative state. How long should biological life be preserved when there is no reasonable prospect of cognitive, sapient life? If the life-support machine is turned off in such circumstances, can this really be considered harmful to the patient, even though the doctor will have terminated a life? Or what about the neurosurgeon who saves a brain-damaged patient from death, only to sentence him to live a life of gross infirmity? Or the doctors who refuse to provide heroic surgery or medical intervention when a child is born suffering from Tay-Sachs disease (spasticity, dementia and death by the age of three or four) or Lesch-Nyhan disease (spasms, mental retardation, compulsive self-mutilation and early death)? Have they really harmed such patients by allowing them to die—or have they saved them from suffering? In other words, when we talk about harm, do we attach more importance to pain and suffering than we do to death itself? Such fine distinctions are not even hinted at in the apparently straightforward proposition, 'above all, do no harm'.

Closely allied to this, of course, is the principle of doing good. It is not enough for doctors not to do harm; they must increase the benefits to others. This means acting in the patient's best interests. But the problem with this is that it is paternalistic. It allows the doctor to decide what is in someone else's best interests without even consulting them. It is based on the assumption that the doctor knows better than anyone, including the patient, what is best for that patient. This brings the principle of beneficence into head-on collision with the next major principle.

Autonomy

The principle of autonomy has become extremely important in our society in a relatively short space of time—certainly since the Second World War and even more recently, within the last twenty years or so. The principle means that individuals should be permitted personal liberty to determine their own actions. Of course, the actual principle of respect for the individual is not new. The concept of the free and sovereign individual was the legacy of John Stuart Mill. His essay, *On Liberty*, was devoted to this one 'very simple principle':

That the only purpose for which power can be rightfully exercised over any member of a civilised community, against his will, is to prevent harm to others. His own good, either physical or moral, is not a sufficient warrant. He cannot rightfully be compelled to do or forbear because it will be better for him to do so, because it will make him happier, because, in the opinions of others, to do so would be wise or even right. These are good reasons for remonstrating with him, or reasoning with him, or persuading him, or entreating him, but not for compelling him or visiting him with any evil in case he do otherwise. To justify that, the conduct from which it is desired to deter him must be calculated to produce evil to someone else. The only part of the conduct or anyone, for which he is amenable to society, is that, which concerns others. In the part which merely concerns himself, his independence is, of right, absolute. Over himself, over his own body and mind the individual is sovereign.

That is, of course, the epigraph for some parts of the world in the second half of the twentieth century. In the UK, this is the era of the sovereign individual, with the law withdrawing from the arena of private morality, with the doctrine of liberty replacing earlier absolute authorities such as God or nature. As Professor Himmelfarb wrote in her introduction to *On Liberty*:

The use and abuse of drugs, crime, punishment, pornography and obscenity, industrial and economic controls, racial and sexual equality, national security and defence, ecology, technology, bureaucracy, education, religion, the family, sex—all come up against the ultimate test: the liberty of the individual. Nor are the most venerable institutions immune to this challenge. It was once only revolutionaries and social rebels who denounced the 'bourgeois' family as authoritarian, ridiculed 'middle-class' notions of sexual normality and morality, declared all social conventions to be incompatible with individuality and condemned all authorities— the state, the law, the church, parents and elders—as agents of coercion. Today, these opinions are the common coin of most liberals.

To her list Professor Himmelfarb might have added medicine. For the challenge to authority, the emphasis on individual rights, has delivered a powerful swipe at the once unquestioned authority of the medical profession. Like other authorities—the church, the family—medicine has seen its very legitimacy questioned. In the widest sense, this has meant a challenge to the principles and organisation of medicine, a charge that it is insular, conservative and may sometimes even do more harm than good. At individual patient level, there is a greater scepticism about the omniscience of doctors and a strong emphasis on patients' rights—for example, in obstetrics, with women campaigning for less doctoring in childbirth, or in mental health, with the Mental Health (Amendment) Act meeting the libertarian critics of the law at least half-way. In fairness, however, it must be pointed out that the conflict is by no means painted in stark black and white. Patients are still, in many cases, happy with or untroubled by paternalism in their doctors; indeed, any physician can cite cases in which the patient wants the doctor to take the burden of decision-making upon his or her own shoulders. And for their part, the medical profession, and the state itself, are not entirely paternalistic. Smoking, for example, is not banned; and most doctors do not refuse to treat patients unless they kick the habit forthwith. Indeed the spectacle of patients who have undergone major and phenomenally expensive heart surgery and then started to smoke again is one which some old-fashioned paternalists can hardly bear!

Truth-telling

This is a principle that is strangely absent from the organised international codes of medical ethics. Strange, because if medical ethics are a bargain between doctors and society, honesty would seem to be fundamental to such a contract. Truthfulness is held to be important both because it is a moral absolute in itself and because, on utilitarian grounds, it produces the best kind of social relationship. Yet medicine's attitude to the truth has always been somewhat ambiguous, mainly because of the way in which it can clash with the

principle of beneficence. Henry Sidgwick has summed it up
in this way:

Where deception is designed to benefit the person deceived,
common sense seems to concede that it may sometimes be right:
for example, most persons would not hesitate to speak falsely to an
invalid, if this seemed the only way of concealing facts that might
produce a dangerous shock. . . . I do not see how we can decide
when and how far it [dishonesty] is admissible, except by
considerations of expediency.

As Robert Veatch has commented, doctors have, by and
large, followed Sidgwick's conclusions:

They have done so, for example, in dealing with terminally ill
patients, and in situations such as genetic counselling where truthfulness might produce harm to the parent being counselled or to the
offspring or in cases in which deception was deemed necessary
to conduct research especially social-psychological research.
Professionals have, on Hippocratic or broader utilitiarian grounds,
supported withholding the truth, deceiving the lay person or even
outright active lying.

There are signs that this is changing, slowly. Doctors are
beginning to tell their patients more. But in general the
question that has to be asked is whether doctors should be the
one group of people in society who are granted an exemption
from a fundamental role of the social game—honesty. As
Veatch comments, this would soon lead to a breakdown of
trust in the lay–professional relationship; no patient would
believe the doctor. And without a perceived honesty on the
part of the doctor, the patient too would inevitably feel that
he or she had the right to lie, or deceive. For this breakdown
of the relationship not to occur, if the doctor is deceiving the
patient, there has to be a double deception—the denial that
the deception is taking place, or the pretence of professional
honesty.

There are, of course, many ways of withholding the truth.
Doctors may use technical jargon to tell someone he has a
terminal illness in an almost subconscious desire simultaneously to tell the truth and to withhold it. Or they may
prevaricate, sàying that they cannot foresee the outcome of

the patient's illness when they actually have a pretty good idea; alternatively, they may paint an over-pessimistic picture, on the grounds that if the patient fares better he will be pleasantly surprised. Any deception of the patient, however, infringes his autonomy or right to know about his condition. The question to be answered is whether that infringement is necessary to observe the other principle of doing good to the patient and not doing harm.

Preserving life
As we have seen already, although existing ethical codes stress the doctor's obligation to respect life, they do not require doctors to preserve life at all costs. This absence of an absolute prohibition opens the way to a number of moral ambiguities. The distinction is drawn, for example, between actively killing a patient and letting that patient die. The former is held to be reprehensible, while the latter is held to be acting in the best interests, sometimes, of the patient. The principle of double effect, already discussed, has similarly evolved through the need to choose between harms. We discuss these controversies in more detail in the chapter on life. At this point, however, what needs to be borne in mind is that the obligation to preserve life may conflict with the obligation to do no harm or to do good. It may also conflict with the patient's own liberty, since by refusing a request to end a suffering patient's life the doctor is overriding the right of that patient to choose death. It might be argued that the patient is still free to commit suicide without the doctor's assistance, and in some cases this may be so. But in others, where the patient is entirely helpless it may not be physically possible for the patient to take his or her own life without the doctor's help. Is the doctor, by refusing to participate in the patient's death, invariably acting in the patient's best interests?

Sometimes he may be; sometimes if the suffering is very great or if the patient is made distressed by the doctor's refusal, the best interests argument becomes more difficult to sustain. In such cases, it seems fair to say that the doctor refuses to participate primarily because to do otherwise would be abhorrent to his own moral codes as an individual and as a doctor, whose role is to heal the sick and not take life. The best interests of the patient would be a secondary consideration.

Justice

The Hippocratic tradition stresses the importance of the doctor's duty towards the individual patient. Taken to extremes, however, this is a socially irresponsible philosophy, since the community is composed of many patients in which care for some may impinge upon the quality of care for others. Complex questions develop about a system of fair distribution as the ethically appropriate way to spread limited resources through the community. This in itself poses problems, since the idea that every individual has a right to health care conflicts with the limited means of society to provide it. Moreover, the needs of some ill people may conflict with the needs of those who are more vulnerable. Take mentally handicapped people, for example, whose needs were ignored for so long. Most people would surely agree that they are entitled to a higher standard of living and thus to a higher level of expenditure. The problem arises when, in a society of limited financial means, the only way to pay for their extra resources is to cut back on care elsewhere. The principle of distributive justice, under which those in greatest need have their needs met first, thus conflicts with the principle of autonomy, under which every individual is entitled to an equal share of the health care provided by the community. If services have to be rationed, how equal can the share-out be? We consider the problems of distributive justice more fully in the chapter on resource allocation.

Religion

The five principles discussed above are the most important ethical absolutes which have somehow to be juggled in a code of modern medical ethics. It may seem a little strange to some people that there has been no mention of organised religion. This is quite deliberate, but should not be understood as an attempt to denigrate the importance of religious ethics to those individuals who practise different faiths. For many people in our society, the moral codes of Roman Catholicism, the Protestant Churches, Judaism or Islam will provide moral guidance in the field of medicine just as they do in other aspects of social life. And the importance generally of what has become known as the Judaeo–Christian tradition in shaping our ethical codes should not be under-estimated. Religious codes of ethics have had their effect on us, the authors of this book, one Jewish and the other influenced by the Church of England, and have imbued us with attitudes that are different from each other's as a result. But while our acquired attitudes may help each of us individually by allowing us to refer to various revealed truths, there is no help there for the development of a collective framework of ethics for medical practice in the United Kingdom. We live in a secular society, and the great majority of doctors and patients will seek the answers to these conundrums within a secular framework.

The limitations of moral philosophy

The distinguished philosopher Professor R.M. Hare wrote in an essay entitled 'Medical ethics: can the moral philosopher help?':

I should like to say at once that if the moral philosopher cannot help with the problems of medical ethics, he ought to shut up shop. The problems of medical ethics are so typical of the moral problems that moral philosophy is supposed to be able to help with, that a failure here really would be a sign either of the uselessness of the discipline or the incompetence of the particular practitioner.

One does not wish to tread too heavily upon such delicate professional sensitivities, but it has to be said that moral philosophy can only make a limited contribution to the problem. Yet the contribution it can and has made should by no means be dismissed. Because medical ethics are, as Professor Hare has said, an example of moral philosophy in action, the subject has become in recent years a kind of adventure playground for philosophers, in which they can be

let loose on equipment to show off their skills within an
environment which is, for them, relatively safe. It is small
wonder that some doctors react with exasperation to such
intellectual gymnastics. The moral philosopher who tells the
paediatrician that there is no moral difference between killing
a handicapped baby and letting it die runs the risk of the
retort that philosophers do not have to make such agonising
decisions daily and under stress; they don't have to confront
traumatised relatives or their own consciences or even,
sometimes, the law. It is a view of philosophy that was well
summed up by Alastair Campbell, a lecturer in Christian
ethics: 'Often, because of its totally abstract and generalised
nature, people either inside or outside the discipline of
philosophy have suspected that 'the Emperor has no clothes';
that because philosophical theories say nothing specific,
they say nothing at all—they are comprehensively, coherent-
ly and lucidly naked!' But as Campbell says, that is an
overstatement of the case. Philosophy is necessary because it
provides us with the means of understanding the problem
and thinking it through in a logical, rational fashion. As
Professor Hare commented:

It is very important, for example, to understand that the relation
between a philosopher and somebody who is troubled about a
question in medical ethics can never be like that between an
old-fashioned general practitioner and his patient. Philosophy is
much more like the teaching of remedial exercises. Philosophers
cannot give their patients pills which the patients can just swallow.
Philosophy itself is the medicine, and it has to be understood, to
some degree at any rate, by the patient himself, in a way that
medical science does not.

In other words, although the paediatrician's irritability
with the philosopher is understandable, there are two
processes at work here which become confused. The first is
the resolution of the philosophical problem of whether or not
allowing a child to die is the same as killing it. It is important
to do this because of the importance we attach to not killing
people. If there is no moral difference between the two, then
we have to understand the moral implications of what we are
doing. In this process, the techniques of philosophical

argument are useful. And it is only when we have resolved that theoretical problem that we can move on to the second process—deciding whether or not such a course of action is right. This is where the philosopher's contribution surely stops. For although he can provide us with the means of discussing the problem, he cannot furnish us with the answer. That is for us to decide—the paediatrician, the parents, society at large. We may say that the doctor would be right to let the child die, even if we have concluded that such an act is no different morally from killing it; or we may say that it must be wrong because there is no difference; or we may say that there is a moral difference and therefore it is permissible. Whatever we say, it is not up to the philosopher to tell us what moral codes to adopt. Philosophy is not a religion, and its practitioners are not priests. Thus, it can only help us to explain and understand the various principles at work in the practice of medicine. It cannot tell us how to resolve the conflicts between them, because at the end of the day someone still has to rank those principles in order of importance, to say that beneficence outweighs autonomy or truth-telling outweighs beneficence, and so on. To expect any more of philosophy will inevitably cause resentment at its failure to provide, as Professor Hare put it, the elixirs of medical ethics. As he said: 'For the true philosopher the most exciting thing in the world—perhaps the only exciting thing—is to become really clear about some important question.' Not, it should be noted, about the answer.

No one argues that medicine should become, or has ever been, a series of *ad hoc* decisions. Medicine has always been governed by broad ethical guidelines within which doctors are free to make individual decisions. The problem is simply that those guidelines are no longer adequate for some problems. In this book, we shall discuss some current medical dilemmas in order to try to illustrate the gap between codes and practice. At the end of the book, we shall try to construct our own tentative list of principles that we think are more suited to the practice of modern medicine. But the underlying questions to be answered are these:

Are the existing ethical mechanisms satisfactory?

If we need ethical codes, who should draft them? What force should they have?

How much discretion should be left to individual doctors in deciding what is right or wrong?

Should any other social institutions, such as the law, have a bearing on medical ethics?

2
LIFE

Behind many of the most agonising dilemmas in modern medicine, behind the emotional and bitter arguments that accompany them, lies the assumption that human life is sacred. The controversies over abortion, post-coital contraception, selective treatment of handicapped babies, euthanasia, *in vitro* fertilisation are all connected by fundamental questions about the importance of life. When does it begin? When does it end? Is life sacred or expendable? Is killing the same as letting die?

Many people—maybe the majority—find these questions too difficult to think about. They are difficult not just because they involve thinking in abstract terms which are hard to define, but because they involve reaching conclusions that are unpalatable. For that reason, they are usually pushed aside and even buried by society at large, only to surface when sensation or scandal attaches to them—the court cases over the care of handicapped babies, for example, or the development of *in vitro* fertilisation. By and large, most people are very happy for doctors, patients and their families to respond to these dilemmas when they arise in their own way, quietly and out of the public gaze. But while each case will always have some unique features, and while doctors must be able to alter their response to the circumstances of an individual case, it cannot be right that the underlying issues should remain a murky area marked 'Do Not Discuss'. Questions about the nature and value of life are the most important moral issues society should face, since they underpin our concept of civilisation. If we do not think about these dilemmas, it is inevitable that inconsistencies will develop and decisions, that will suit no one, will be taken in a vacuum. We talk about 'rights' in this book and by that we

21

mean a claim that has been granted by the society in which a person lives. It is an animal urge to want to live and in normal circumstances an animal will choose a course of action that will tend to preserve its life. An animal that is attacked and threatened will try to defend itself. We believe, as a premise for this chapter, that *all* human beings make a claim to life. The questions that we consider are about the circumstances in which that claim is granted the status of a 'right'.

Is life sacred?

Most of us think that killing someone is wrong and abhorrent. It is the worst crime we can commit and we reserve for it the most draconian sanctions in our society. We think it is wrong both for absolute and utilitarian reasons. The utilitarian reasons are far easier to explain. Killing people causes pain and unhappiness; moreover, if the value of life were not upheld, civilised order would rapidly descend into chaos. But our revulsion against killing goes deeper than this. We feel it offends against some absolute code of morality. This view was famously articulated by Albert Schweitzer, who wrote:

I cannot but have reverence for all that is called life. I cannot avoid compassion for all that is called life. This is the beginning and foundation of morality. . . . Ethics thus consists in this, that I experience the necessity of practising the same reverence for life toward all will–to–live as toward my own. Therein I have already the needed fundamental principle of morality. It is good to maintain and cherish life; it is evil to destroy and check life.

Schweitzer clearly chose to grant a person's claim to life in any and every case. Indeed, it's probable that he would have considered the question intolerably presumptuous. The same view was even more strongly expressed by Edward Shils:

To persons who are not murderers, concentration camp administrators or dreamers of sadistic fantasies, the inviolability of human life seems to be so self-evident that it might appear pointless to inquire into it. To inquire into it is embarrassing as well because, once raised, the question seems to commit us to beliefs we do not wish to espouse and to confront us with contradictions which seem to deny what is self-evident.

To which the response of anyone who thinks about this for a second must be, 'Yes, but . . .'. For the contradictions are all around us. Unless we are pacifists, for example, we accept that it is proper to take life in wartime, or in self-defence. Even organised religions, which many assume embody the doctrine of the sanctity of life, do not hold that it is an absolute doctrine. The Roman Catholic Church, for example, states that it is not necessary to use 'extraordinary means' to prolong life. Even Judaism, which places a higher value on human life than the Christian tradition, and which regards human life as sacred from the formation of the sperm to the decomposition of the body, permits abortion when the foetus is threatening the mother's life, on the grounds that the foetus, although a form of life, has not been granted the same rights as a newborn baby or the mother.

So whether we hold secular humanist or religious views, it seems that the sanctity of life is not an absolute value, one that is inviolable in any circumstances. There are some circumstances in which we hold that it may be overriden by other, conflicting, moral considerations that we consider to be more important. During the Nazi period in Germany, there were some doctors who, in the knowledge that their helplessly hospitalised patients were about to be abused or murdered or transported to concentration camps, made poison available to them or even administered fatal doses to them without their knowledge in order to spare them from the horrors that awaited them. Who would say that such doctors were acting unethically? So it becomes an ethically tenable position to say that human life may not be sacred, but it is extremely important. This does not tell us, though, why we think it is important, what it is about life that we value.

For religious believers, the issue is relatively straightforward. Life is valuable because it is God-given; human life is especially valuable because of the possession of an immortal soul. It is not for mortals to question who should enjoy the right to life. These are matters of faith, not susceptible to logical explanation. But for the non-believer, the secular humanist, the question is more difficult to answer. Does human life have intrinsic value—or is it valuable only for subsidiary characteristics it may possess? Even those who hold no overt religious beliefs often say that life is intrinsically valuable. Thus they would not disconnect the positive pressure ventilator or life-support machine from a patient in an irreversible coma. On the other hand, there are those who believe that life has no intrinsic value. The philosopher Jonathan Glover, for example, has argued that neither life nor 'mere' consciousness are valuable in themselves but because they are necessary for other things that matter in themselves. These things, he says, are the ingredients of 'a life worth living'. He doesn't, however, specify what those ingredients are; indeed, he concedes that he cannot do so, for the best judge of the worth of a life must be the person living it. In so doing, he concedes that the principle of autonomy is more important than the utilitarian values of a worthwhile life. Indeed, the principle of autonomy is crucial to those humanists who feel that life is intrinsically valuable. For a start, the utilitarian argument is dangerous. This is because it appears to follow, once we have decided that someone's life is unhappy or useless or damaging to the rest of the community, that such a life should be ended. People who were thought to contribute little to the well-being of society should be considered replaceable. Utilitarianism holds that killing is wrong if it increases the stock of misery and diminishes the stock of happiness; does it follow that utilitarians would think it right to kill people with low utility so that more people could be added with higher utility. As Sheila MacLean and Gerry Maher have argued, they could say that:

persons of socio-economic class 4 or 5 or who belong to certain racial or religious minority groups have not the remotest chance of enjoying a happy life or adding to the overall social happiness. And given certain assumptions about what constitutes a happy life, this conclusion might in one sense be true, for we do think that certain people have fewer 'chances' than others (say the children of a poor immigrant family as opposed to children of a well-off middle-class family). Such assessments are a common feature of the thinking of the sort of society in which we live. The only counter-consideration which utilitarianism can offer is to point to the threat to the general security of society if such reasoning were accepted, but any such consequences are merely contingent and they may not exist in some situations as where minorities are easily identifiable and can be distinguished from others. What is the weakest aspect of utilitarianism, then, is that it gives no scope for consideration of the interests of an individual person as these appear to the particular person concerned.

This philosophy is repugnant because it conflicts with our strong sense of the rights of the individual, or, to use the jargon again, the person's autonomy. As MacLean and Maher point out, this respect for autonomy goes far beyond the practical point that the best way to discover the values important to someone is to leave the decision to that person.

Autonomy theories, however, argue that humans have special moral attributes, most notably their ability to understand and act upon moral rules (the idea of self-determination). Indeed, this is what makes them persons. Moreover, these theories hold that moral rules must apply to everyone and we must respect everyone's right to self-determination if we concede his or her moral standing. Thus, in deciding upon a person's continued existence without having regard to his own views, we infringe the most basic moral principle of respect for persons as ends in themselves.

In other words, even for the utilitarian, there is a basis for believing in the intrinsic value of human life—the belief that every individual in a society has rights, and among those rights is the right to life. But that does not resolve the problems in medical practice. For a start, non-pacifists would not accept the claim that all individuals have an absolute right to life. Even the 'pro-Life' campaigners against the British abortion law would probably support a 'just' war or self-defence. Most people who support an individual's right to life would take the view that it is a prima facie right, and that we should act on the presumption that killing is wrong—although in certain circumstances, a greater potential wrong might mean that the wrong of killing is permissible. Secondly, it does not guide us in situations when the autonomy of the patient cannot be expressed—for example, in cases involving unborn children, newborn babies, the senile or otherwise mentally infirm patient, and those in a coma. Such people can make no choices and are unaware of their rights.

So we conclude that people do have an intrinsic right to life, a claim that should be granted, although this is not an absolute right and may be overridden in certain circumstances. Life, in other words, is not absolutely inviolable. This uncertain doctrine is embodied in medical codes of practice and generally in the organisation of our society. The Hippocratic Oath, for example, contains no reference to preserving the sanctity of life as such, although it does prohibit the giving of deadly medicine or a pessary to produce abortion. The Declaration of Geneva says: 'I will maintain the utmost respect for human life from the time of conception . . . A doctor must always bear in mind the obligation of preserving human life.' This statement falls far short of an explicit instruction always to preserve life in any circumstances. Medical codes could not contain such an explicit instruction, since as we shall see later in this chapter there are occasions where a doctor's duty to prevent suffering, for example, conflicts with his obligation to preserve life.

In our society we do not assume that life has to be preserved at all costs. We would not throw someone under a bus; nor would we stand idly by while someone threw himself under the bus. But we know that while there are buses, there is a danger that people will be killed in accidents involving them, and yet we do not ban buses. Instead, we calculate that the general good to society in having a bus service outweighs the occasional disasters that such a service might bring, including a possible loss of life. An organised society would be impossible if we did not make, implicitly or explicitly, such calculations. When such calculations are translated into public policy, however, we may object because we feel that life should not come with a price tag. For example, some years ago an interdepartmental working group on smoking concluded that the cost to the country of a massive drop in smoking would be unacceptable, since apart from factors such as the loss of jobs in the cigarette industry, the greater number of people surviving into pensionable age would impose too great a strain upon the Exchequer. This was greeted with some revulsion as an example of the cynicism of Whitehall in deciding that the lives of British citizens were simply too expensive. It is an example of the utilitarian argument about the value of human life at work, and a demonstration of how that philosophy can overrule the notion that people have rights (in this case, to health and life).

But however repugnant this particular example may have been, it is a fact that decisions are made all the time in public circles which assume that human life is not sacred, not absolutely inviolable and not to stand in the way of a presumed greater good. The basis upon which such decisions should be made is intensely problematic, not least in medicine, where the boundaries of life are subject to intense debate.

When does life begin?

This simple question is extremely difficult to answer. If we could answer it neatly, and in a way which would command everyone's agreement, medical decision-making would become far easier. Some commentators, unable to resolve the issue in a satisfactory way, have concluded that there is little point in trying to establish the answer to the question. What does it matter when life begins, they argue, since what is important is the quality of the human state. This approach works well for those who do not believe that life itself has intrinsic value. For those who do believe it has such value, that it possesses an essential dignity which should command our respect, it is necessary to work out what we're actually talking about. If we don't want to harm or destroy life, then we have to determine its boundaries. The trouble is that the start of life, the boundary at the beginning, is not a provable scientific fact; it is a matter of philosophical interpretation or religious belief which differs from person to person.

It is currently fashionable to say that life does not begin at all. Rather, it continues from generation to generation; it does not spring up afresh in every individual, but is passed down in a continuous chain of evolution. Certainly, it is hard to deny this when life in its broadest sense is considered to mean existence on this planet. But this attitude is not particularly helpful in everyday medical decision-making. We may agree that our individual lives are part of a continuing process, but few of us would seriously contend that a foetus is simply a bundle of cells growing inside the body, an appendage to the mother of no more significance than, say, a wart.

It is extremely difficult to identify the point at which a foetus achieves the right to life. For Roman Catholics, there is no problem. From the moment of conception there exists a person with a soul. For supporters of abortion on demand, the foetus is simply a part of the mother's body and it is her right to decide what to do with it. The Roman Catholic approach is a matter of faith and therefore brooks no argument—you either believe it, or you don't. The abortion on demand argument, however, is flawed in a different way since presumably even its most passionate adherents would draw the line at aborting a foetus because it had, say, red hair or brown eyes. There would surely be a repugnance against such an act, and such repugnance is not explained by the 'life is a continuum' argument alone. It is presumably explained by the recognition of the claim to life exerted by the growth inside the mother's body. When does that claim arise and upon what is it founded? Is the foetus a person? A potential person? A life form? And at what stage in the reproductive process has it gained this dignity?

It helps to look in some detail at the various stages at which life has been deemed to begin. For some, it begins at birth. The attractions of this approach are obvious. There can be no doubt at birth that a human being exists, recognisable as a tiny individual and capable of independent existence, provided it is given warmth and food. But the demarcation of birth is inadequate, because it does not dispose of the possibility that before birth, for a period of days or even weeks, it had reached such a stage of development that if—hypothetically—it had been lifted out of its mother's uterus it would have survived just as well. Indeed, there have been disturbing cases where late abortions have produced living babies. And as Roger Wertheimer has written, if mothers had transparent wombs we would certainly regard the foetus in its later stages of development at least as a living creature, even if it was not yet living an independent life. It seems that the birth demarcation argument rests on a self-deception caused by the fact that the foetus is not visible.

For a long time, individual existence was held to begin at quickening, the moment when the mother feels the foetal movements for the first time. This, however, has no significance at all for the development of the foetus. Modern English law chooses another point in its development to draw the boundary—viability or the point at which a baby can survive independently of the mother. This, however, is an administrative convenience rather than a moral certainty. The time at which viability occurs depends upon the medical expertise that is available to help a baby to live if it is delivered at this boundary. As medical skills develop so the boundary moves further back, but only for babies born where the expertise and equipment is available. So if viability were adopted as a boundary of human life, we would have the absurd situation in which life began in America, say, at 22 weeks gestation but in Ethiopia at 34 weeks. Or, as Jonathan Glover puts it, '. . . we might say "last year this foetus would not have been a person at this stage, but since they re-equipped the intensive care unit, it is one." '

Another administrative convenience is the use of implantation as the boundary to define the beginning of life. The argument here is that it is only when the fertilised egg embeds itself in the mother's body that life begins, for it is only then that the egg has the means of realising its potential and developing into a baby. But this argument, deployed by the Department of Health and Social Security, and so apparently seductive, won't do. For a start, it might not be long before scientists develop an artificial placenta to sustain an embryo outside the womb. (Devotees of the implantation boundary, however, might plausibly argue that this would make no difference in principle, since it could still be argued that because the embryo needs sustenance in order to develop, the point at which it was joined to the artificial placenta would be the beginning of life.) But there seems to be a more fundamental argument against this boundary. To say that life does not exist because it has no means of sustaining its development is a *non sequitur*. If a newborn baby were abandoned in a cold street with inadequate clothing and no food, it would surely die within a short space of time; but we would not therefore say that the baby had never existed as an independent individual. So it is with the fertilised egg. Just because it is undeniably true that the fertilised egg would not survive if it were not implanted, it does not necessarily follow at all that the fertilised egg before implantation does not fit the definition of life.

This leads us to the last and most important boundary—conception. This is the boundary set by Roman Catholics—among others—and which, if accepted, would mean that abortion or the squashing of foetuses conceived by *in vitro* fertilisation involves the destruction of human life. The arguments against this boundary are hard to support. Indeed, they are often characterised by a confusion of thinking. For example, it is said that the fertilised egg cannot be called a person because it is so unlike us. But few people would call the embryo at this stage in its development a person; what it undeniably is, however, is a potential person. But saying that the fertilised egg is not a person, only a potential person, is not the same as saying that it is not human life, only potential human life. Becoming a person is a gradual process involving the emergence of consciousness, the ability to form relationships, to have emotional responses, to have a sense of identity, and so on. Obviously the foetus has none of these characteristics, but it is incontestably a potential person. It has a claim to life.

It is also a form of actual life, in a way that the unfertilised egg or the sperm are not. This is because the fertilised egg is a single cell with a complete set of chromosomes, as opposed to the unfertilised egg or the sperm which have only half the required number of chromosomes. The fertilised egg, therefore, all other things being equal (which, it has to be said, often they are not) will divide and develop. The unfertilised human egg or sperm will not. It may be that the day will arrive when a human embryo can be formed by parthenogenesis, just as we know now that frogs' eggs can be induced to double their chromosomes without being fertilised. If that were ever to happen, it would mean that human life had been created, albeit by artificial means. But until that happens, the unfertilised human egg cannot be considered as life, since it cannot develop.

If the fertilised ovum is a potential human being, then because it is an individual with a unique genetic make-up, it deserves our respect. This is because of our belief, stated earlier, in the principle of autonomy and the rights of an individual, including the right to life. But there are some who claim that the principle of autonomy cannot apply to babies. Jonathan Glover, for example, argues: 'Since unfertilised eggs, foetuses and newborn babies are all without even the capacity for any desire for life, they all fall outside the scope of the principle of autonomy.' Apart from lumping together unfertilised ova and newborn babies, this appears to be a most dangerous argument. What about an old person suffering from senile dementia, or other mentally ill or handicapped people who may not be able to think in these terms? If we do not recognise such people's claim to life then this would seem to be a fast route to the concentration camps. Babies are people; unborn babies are potential people. All are intensely vulnerable precisely because they cannot articulate that claim to life that most of us would allow them to have.

When does life end?

In the past, this question has been a source of considerable controversy, created as a result of advances in medical science. Until recently, death was a simple state to identify, since respiration and heart-beat would stop and from then on the body would start to decompose. However, advances in our understanding of biochemistry and physiology, and the introduction of artificial respiration, or intermittent positive pressure ventilation changed this dramatically.

In the majority of cases death is not a discrete, immediate event but a process in which the various organs cease to function at different times. Sometimes, death occurs instantaneously or nearly instantaneously as a result óf, say, a massive heart attack. But with developments in resuscitation and life support, it is now possible to keep the heart and respiratory functions going even when there is little likelihood of an individual recovering consciousness after massive brain damage. The Conference of Royal Medical Colleges said in a Memorandum in 1979:

It is now universally accepted, by the lay public as well as by the medical profession, that it is not possible to equate death itself with the cessation of the heart beat. Quite apart from the elective cardiac arrest of open-heart surgery, spontaneous cardiac arrest followed by successful resuscitation is today a commonplace and although the more sensational accounts of occurrences of this kind still refer to the patient being 'dead' until restoration of the heart beat, the use of the quote marks usually demonstrates that this word is not to be taken literally, for to most people the one aspect of death that is beyond debate is its irreversibility.

Much of the controversy over the definition of death appears to have been the result of some muddled thinking. Brain-stem death has become the most satisfactory definition of death because if the brain-stem has ceased to function, the brain cannot function at all. After death of the brain-stem has occurred, the regulating mechanisms of the body fail and it is merely a matter of time before the body starts to decompose. This is not the same as the kind of severe cerebral brain-damage which produces an irreversible coma, and in which the patient is capable of maintaining homeostasis. The patient (Karen Quinlan, for example) is still alive by this definition, albeit in a vegetative state.

Brain-stem death has been inadequately understood and there have been fears that it is a way of hurrying death along. There has been particular concern, for example, over cases in which a patient is said to be brain-stem dead and his organs are removed for transplantation while his heart is still beating. The definition of death as being an irreversible cessation of function in the brain-stem can be a means of allowing a patient to die with dignity and of sparing his relatives unnecessary distress—provided it is explained to them. Misapprehensions have arisen through inadequate explanation. For example, wrong diagnoses made in the past have led some to believe that recovery from death of the brain-stem is possible, when it is not; and provided the established criteria are observed, such mistakes should not happen. Similarly, there was some question in a recent murder case about whether the defendant had been responsible for the victim's death since it was the doctors at the hospital who had actually turned off the ventilator. What was not appreciated was that the victim's brain-stem was already dead, so the loss of the ventilator was neither here nor there. Indeed, had the ventilator not been turned off, the body would have started to rot. Whether this inevitability is widely understood is open to some doubt.

There is, however, another controversy over the definition of death. This concerns those people whose brain-stems are not dead but whose brains are nevertheless so badly damaged that they are doomed to remain indefinitely comatose. Glover discusses the argument that such people are actually dead:

Two candidates sometimes proposed are that 'death' should be defined in terms of the irreversible loss of all electrical activity in the brain or that it should be defined in terms of irreversible loss of consciousness. Of these two definitions, the one in terms of irreversible loss of consciousness is preferable. There is no point in considering the electrical activity unless one holds the (surely correct) view that it is a necessary condition of the person being conscious.

But he then goes on to admit that in ordinary language it makes sense to say of someone that he is irreversibly comatose but still alive:

The proposed account of death is a piece of conceptual revision, motivated by the belief that, for such purposes as deciding whether or not to switch off a respirator, the irreversibly comatose and the traditionally 'dead' are on a par.

What Glover seems to be saying is not that the irreversibly comatose person is dead, but that the quality of that life is so poor that we should end it. Suppose for a moment that we should, although there would seem to be serious arguments against this, most notably that we should not kill people. If we were to do so, however, we should be sure about what we were doing—that it was killing an individual, and this should never be confused with officiating at a death that had already spontaneously occurred.

Killing and letting die

Is letting die the same as killing? This is a question beloved of moral philosophers and loathed by those doctors who are faced in their daily practice by the need to choose between prolonging a life of misery and allowing it to end. Such doctors say that to argue about such fine distinctions—which they concede are narrow—is a luxury to be afforded only by academics and others who never have to confront a baby with a frightful handicap or its distraught parents. Such doctors deserve our sympathy and admiration. They do what they do from the highest motives, whether they take an absolutist line that they must preserve the lives of handicapped children or whether they choose to let some die. But however elevated their motives, the implications of what they are doing have to be faced. If letting someone die is morally no different from killing, then we should be clear about what we are doing.

There are, as we shall see, circumstances in which doctors allow their patients to die. Yet doctors argue passionately that there is a difference betwen allowing patients to die and killing them—not just a practical but a moral difference. Even those doctors who say that morally there is little to choose between killing and letting die are emphatic that they might withdraw treatment but they would never kill. In the main, advances in medical technology and skills have benefited society. People who would otherwise have died from, say, a heart attack have been reprieved from death through improvements in resuscitation techniques. Premature babies, or those born with serious disabilities who would otherwise have died at birth are being saved routinely in special care baby units.

But there is a darker side to these advances. Because medical science can now save life so effectively, it is sometimes able to fend off death only to expose the patient to continuing misery and suffering. Thus, a doctor's duty to respect life and preserve it wherever possible comes into direct conflict with his duty to prevent and relieve pain. The Hippocratic Oath set out the duty: 'The regimen I adopt shall be for the benefit of the patients according to my ability and judgment, and not for their hurt or for any wrong.' This concept is more generally recognised as the maxim *primum non nocere*—above all, do no harm—which most doctors regard as an absolute principle above all others, including the duty to preserve life. As Dr R.I.S. Bayliss wrote in a British Medical Journal leading article in 1982: 'In medical ethics, life is not the absolute good, nor death the absolute evil. Not to harm the patient (primum non nocere) has Hippocratic origins. To restore health or relieve suffering does not imply that it is ethically right to prolong life at any cost.'

The distinction between doing something and allowing something to happen is built into our society's codes. Murdering someone is considered far worse than standing watching the murder being committed. A distinction is drawn between an act and an omission. Similarly, the doctrine of double effect is widely accepted. Broadly this means that although it is always wrong intentionally to do a bad act for the sake of good consequences that will ensue, it may be right to do a good act in the knowledge that bad consequences will ensue. So, for example, if a pregnant woman has cancer of the uterus, it would be right to remove the uterus even though this would mean the death of the foetus.

If these principles were not adhered to the doctors would be committed to unreservedly using every skill and resource to try to save every single life that presents to them, an impossible instruction. As Philippa Foot has commented:

most of us allow people to die of starvation in India and Africa and

there is surely something wrong with us that we do; it would be
nonsense, however, to pretend that it is only in law that we make a
distinction between allowing people in the underdeveloped countries to die of starvation and sending them poisoned food.

Critics of these doctrines argue, however, that the distinctions are specious because the consequences are identical.
Thus, the foetus in the cancerous uterus dies anyway,
regardless of whether the death was willed. The starving
millions in India and Africa will die anyway, regardless of the
fact that we have not actually poisoned them.

At the level of personal medical care the dilemma does not
present a significant problem when the patient is able to say
for himself whether he wishes his doctor to prolong his life
or to allow him to die. If a patient does not want treatment, it
is his right to make such a decision. (A difficulty here
concerns the doctor's duty when the patient wants active
assistance with his own death, and we shall consider this
later.) The trouble arises when the patient is not competent to
make such a decision, for example in cases involving
newborn babies or sufferers from senile dementia. The
doctor is then in a most difficult position, since he is faced
with a series of unanswerable questions.

Who should decide whether the patient's life is too awful
to be saved? With newborn infants, doctors stress that such
decisions are made after the most careful consultation with
the parents and consideration of their wishes. But this does
not solve the problem of the doctor's duty. For a start,
parents in such circumstances are probably distressed beyond
measure, maybe unable to think straight, maybe prone to
make decisions they will later regret; even if they are calm
and composed, they will probably be disproportionately
influenced by what the doctor tells them. If they decide that
the baby should not be helped to live, the doctor cannot
escape the fact that he then has to decide where his duty
lies—to preserve that life or to allow it to snuff out. So how
does he take that decision? Whose interests should he
consider, since he may well be faced with competing interests
between the patient, the family and society at large? How
does he measure the quality of the patient's life? How great

does the actual or prospective pain and suffering have to be before he decides to allow the child to die?

These are terrible questions, and as yet society has come up with no satisfactory answers. Indeed, society has not yet faced up to the challenge of trying to think such issues through to produce consistent guidelines. So inconsistencies abound, and doctors are left to flounder in an uneasy legal limbo, looking over their shoulders all the time at the activities of the religious vigilante squads who have set themselves up as society's unauthorised policemen of doctors' ethical behaviour.

Some instances of selective non-treatment are relatively uncontroversial. For instance, most people would agree that the actual process of dying should not be prolonged unnecessarily—the prolonged death of President Tito and General Franco demonstrated how a medical refusal to bow to the inevitable can rob the dying patient of his dignity. The difficulty arises most acutely, however, when the desire not to fight the inevitable becomes confused with terminating or withholding treatment because of a questionable value judgement. For example, it would be wrong to refuse to treat an otherwise hale 80-year-old for pneumonia when that person might, if treated, recover and live for another ten years in contentment. But if the 80-year-old had senile dementia and not a relative in the world, then a good case could be made for saying that it would be kinder to step back and let pneumonia assume its traditional role as the old person's friend.

Similarly, most people would agree that it would be wrong to prolong the life of a baby born with its brain outside its head. But there is considerable disagreement about other forms of handicap. Professor Alastair Campbell argued in 1982:

Many paediatricians would probably agree that the most important medical criterion is severe abnormality, disease or damage to the central nervous system, especially the brain, which will have devastating consequences for development. If there is little prospect of freedom from crippling disabilities that will prevent the attainment of a personal life of meaning and quality, and a measure

of independence from others, then extraordinary means to sustain
or prolong life are inappropriate. Specific examples include infants
with severe microcephaly, severe neural tube defects, gross
hydrocephalus if complicated by infection, and chromosomal
disorders such as Trisomy 13 and 18. Infants with extensive and
fully documented (by clinical and imaging criteria) brain damage
after asphyxia and haemorrhage might also be included.

An honest response to the dilemma was put forward by
Professor John Lorber in his case for the selective treatment
of spina bifida babies, quoted by John Harris in a paper in
1981. Lorber wrote: 'It is essential that nothing should be
done which might prolong the infant's survival', and that the
temptation to operate should be resisted because 'progressive
hydrocephalus is an important cause of early death'. Those
who support Professor Lorber's policy of selective treatment
do so because of the terrible suffering such children would
otherwise undergo. But there have been several examples of
spina bifida sufferers writing indignantly to the newspapers
and other journals to point out that despite their grave
handicaps they live enjoyable and worthwhile lives which
they would not have wanted to forgo.

There appears to be no valid moral distinction to be drawn
between allowing such babies to die and killing them—which
leads Harris and others to argue inexorably for infanticide, on
the grounds that if one wants a baby to die, it would be more
humane to put the child and the family out of their misery as
quickly as possible. And on simple, logical grounds, it does
seem impossible to argue against this attitude. Lorber, for
example, does not try to argue against the logic but uses
other powerful practical arguments instead—such as the
danger of brutalisation, the fact that if babies were actually
killed the trauma for parents and staff would be insupport-
able and far greater than the trauma involved in allowing
them to die. Arguments like these undoubtedly carry great
weight in themselves, and may by themselves be sufficient to
prevent a policy of infanticide from being implemented. But
we have to recognise that we have progressively undermined
the strongest moral argument against infanticide.
Beauchamp and Childress, for example, argue that permit-

ting active killing would mean a general reduction of respect for human life. 'Rules against killing in a moral code are not isolated moral principles; they are threads in a fabric of rules that support respect for human life. The more threads we remove, the weaker the fabric becomes.' But threads have already been removed from that fabric, and doctors and others delude themselves if they do not recognise that fact. As the *BMJ* argued in 1981:

Within the space of a single generation termination of pregnancy has become accepted as routine when the foetus is at high risk of mental or physical defect (though opinion is much more divided on the 'social' indications for abortion). Critics of the Abortion Act 1967 warned that it might pave the way for euthanasia of handicapped infants. They were right—to some extent—for severely handicapped infants are now seen by many doctors and parents as having less than an absolute claim to every possible form of medical treatment.

It may well be that developments such as legal abortion and the selective treatment of handicapped babies are desirable and necessary, however difficult it proves to determine the criteria for such decisions. But this should not blind us to the slope down which we have slid so far and the direction in which we are still slipping. It is all very well for doctors and others to uphold with passion the distinction between killing and letting die, justifying the latter but resisting the former; but thirty years ago or less, they would probably have found the idea that doctors would decide not to use standard procedures to save the life of a Down's Syndrome baby as outlandish and repugnant as anything dreamed up by Aldous Huxley. We may conclude that it is in the interests of society to carry on down this route, but in doing so we cannot ignore the unpalatable fact that we are all the time eroding our respect for life.

Another set of related dilemmas concerns neither the very old, nor the newborn but those who have suffered brain damage. Mr Sam Galbraith, a Scottish neurosurgeon, has said that such dilemmas arise out of what he calls 'the no-lose philosophy of medicine'. By this, he means that doctors will prescribe drugs or a respirator for a patient even though they know this is useless—on the basis that they can't lose anything by doing so, and might just possibly gain some benefit. Thus patients with severe head injuries are vigorously treated but may end up as human vegetables. Ethics, he says, have become confused with mathematics. What matters is the number of lives saved, when what should matter is the quality of the lives saved.

This goes to the crux of the dilemma. If we accept, as most of us do, that an absolute commitment to save life at all costs is untenable, then we have to accept that we have replaced a commitment to preserving the sanctity of life by a commitment to upholding the quality of life. But who is to decide what quality should be supported and what should be considered dispensable? What criteria should be used? The patient's social worth? The disproportionate cost to society? Such criteria would be tantamount to creating a super-race in which ill-functioning or non-productive people are cast aside. This would be quite unacceptable (although, as we shall show, we are coming perilously close to that point). A more acceptable criterion is one which balances the pain and suffering of the individual against the values he can derive from his life. However great the burden on society, however punishing the pressure on the family, the decision should be taken from the point of view of the patient's own interests. And in deciding what is best for those interests, it would also be wrong to be influenced by the fear that social conditions for the patient might be less than hospitable. Just because there is a possibility that a handicapped child might end up in an institution, this should not mean that less care is spent in preserving that child's life, just as it would be wrong to allow an old person to die simply because of the poor quality of life in the old people's home. These are administrative, social or political concerns and should not impinge on the question of whether a life is worth living.

Several commentators have understandably argued that the criteria governing such decisions should be drawn as tightly as possible. One commentator who has sought to define the indefinable is Ian Kennedy, the lawyer and Reith lecturer. He proposed that the criterion should be 'the capacity to flourish as a human being', but this would also seem to pose more questions than it answered. How would we define 'flourish', for example, or even more problematically, 'as a human being'? But the impetus behind these quests for definition is understandable and right. As Kennedy says, 'We must ensure that the class of those marked for death is kept as narrowly and strictly defined as possible'. The need for society at large to address itself to these issues and formulate such a code, rather than leave such decisions to evolve in an *ad hoc* manner, was emphasised by two important court cases in 1981. These cases, both concerning the treatment of newly-born Down's Syndrome babies, demonstrated the confusion and inconsistencies that all of us, doctors, judges, juries, have allowed to develop in this under-exposed area. They also served as a perhaps timely warning that, in the absence of a generally acceptable set of standards worked out by society at large, we have slid further down this particular slope, perhaps, than we might have wished.

The case of Alexandra

Alexandra was a Down's Syndrome baby born with an intestinal blockage which would have killed her if it had not been operated upon. Her distressed parents decided it would be best not to operate but to let her die, since nature appeared to have 'made its own arrangements to terminate a life which could not be fruitful'. The doctor would not operate without their consent. The case was referred to the local social services department, which applied to court to overturn the parents' decision, which the Court of Appeal eventually did, thus authorising the surgery to go ahead. The case was notable because it reaffirmed that parents are not entitled to choose death for their children. It also laid down that it was in the best interests of the child to live, which was a decision that seemed entirely right. Down's Syndrome children can often grow up into adults who, although handicapped, live lives of serenity and enjoyment. The quality of their lives is not unbearably awful, as it may be with spina bifida babies or with children with other multiple handicaps. A normal child with an intestinal blockage would unquestionably have a

correcting operation, so the only reason for withholding
surgery in this case would have been the result of a value
judgement about the quality of a Down's child's life. And
since the presumption must have been that Alexandra could
look forward to 20 or 30 years of relatively untroubled life, it
seemed that the parents' decision had more to do with their
own inability to come to terms with their handicapped child,
or their ignorance of her prospects, or both, than it did with
her best interests.

The case of Dr Arthur

The judgment of the Court of Appeal in the Alexandra case,
which upheld the principle of the child's autonomy, appeared
to conflict with the decision of the jury in the Arthur case,
which appeared to uphold the antithetical principle of
paternalism, or the doctor's right to decide on behalf of his
patient. (One has to be a little cautious about drawing too
many conclusions from the Arthur case because a criminal
trial, conducted on an accusatorial basis, is not designed to
establish the truth but to establish guilt or innocence; and the
reasons why the jury acquitted Dr Arthur remain among the
secrets of the jury room.) The facts of the case are these. Dr
Leonard Arthur, a senior consultant paediatrician at Derby
City Hospital, was called in to examine a newly-born
Down's Syndrome baby. The parents were very distressed,
and Dr Arthur made a note: 'Parents do not wish it to
survive. Nursing care only.' He prescribed a sedative drug,
dihydrocodeine, to alleviate distress as and when it arose.
Three days later the baby died, and the cause of death was
given as bronchopneumonia due to consequences of Down's
Syndrome. Dr Arthur was then charged with murder, with
the prosecution alleging that he had prescribed the sedative in
order to kill the child and that the child had further been
deprived of food and medical treatment so that it would die.
The prosecution's case fell apart at the seams, however, when
it was revealed that the baby had further defects in his heart,
lungs and brain which could have been the cause of death. So
the charge was changed to one of attempted murder, with the
prosecution attempting to prove that even if he hadn't caused
the baby's death, he had intended to do so. The defence

maintained that, as the law and paediatric practice permit, Dr Arthur had instead simply allowed nature to take its course. Dr Arthur was acquitted.

Since the prosecution had so clearly failed to do its homework properly, there is a strong argument for saying that Dr Arthur should never have been put in the dock. But since he was, the case was an important one since, in the vacuum created by the lack of any public discussion about these matters, it provided a rare opportunity for the public to hear from a number of distinguished doctors about prevalent attitudes in good paediatric practice. For example, Dr Peter Dunn, a paediatrician, said:

Some children are born with such frightful handicaps that we think it is reasonable to accept the parents' decision that in the interest of their own child, prolonging, or long life is not in that interest. It is an extremely complex matter. No paediatrician takes life; but we accept that allowing babies to die—and I know the distinction is narrow but we all feel it tremendously profoundly—is in the baby's interest at times.

As we have already seen, few would disagree with that as a general principle. The difficulty about the Arthur case was, though, that here was a baby with Down's Syndrome but who—to the parents and doctors treating him, at least—suffered from no additional handicap or illness. (The internal ailments were only discovered in the post-mortem examination.) So while it would seem perfectly reasonable to sedate a baby in distress, even if the side-effect of that sedation might be to suppress appetite and so hasten death, it was never explained why such a sedative was needed in this case. Secondly, and again from the point of view of the doctors at the time, the baby was apparently healthy despite its handicap; there was no reason to suppose that, like baby Alexandra, it might not look forward to many years of reasonable life. If such a 'normal' Down's baby contracted an infection and was not treated, the only reason he would not be treated was that he was mentally handicapped. Since Down's Syndrome is, as we have said, a form of mental handicap that might not prevent the sufferer from living a reasonable life, it would seem that this particular value

judgement would be based not on the best interests of the
patient and the quality of his life but on other, external
factors—distress to the family, for instance, or maybe even
the burden to society. While the family's distress, and the
damage to the family unit that may be caused by such a birth
should not be under-estimated, such considerations surely
should not affect a decision to withhold treatment. It is hard
to see how such a decision could square with any codes of
medical ethics.

The judge in the Arthur case said in his instructions to the
jury that it was lawful to treat babies with sedating drugs and
offer no food or surgery if certain criteria were met—that the
child must be irreversibly disabled, and rejected by its
parents. This would appear to conflict with the judgment in
the Alexandra case, which held that the parents' rejection
should not cause the child's death; a decision to allow a child
to die should only be made when it was in the child's best
interests. The judge in the Arthur case seemed to be implying
that a baby did not have any rights independent of its parents.
Secondly, the other criterion, that the child must be
irreversibly disabled, cannot be right. It makes no mention of
the severity of the disability, or the capacity of the child to
function as a human being in spite of its disability. As we
have said, such definitions are notoriously difficult to make,
but Mr Justice Farquharson's attempt seems to have little to
commend it ethically, not to mention having left the law in a
mess.

The question remains of who, if anyone, should try to
construct such criteria to impose some degree of consistency.
The British Paediatric Association has made no attempt to do
this. Its members have decided, for example, that the
instruction 'nursing care only', which is capable of varying
interpretations, should mean giving a baby food, warmth
and love—the basic requirements of any normal baby. But
the BPA also cannot escape the contradictions of these cases.
For instance, it has said that 'a malformed infant has the same
rights as a normal infant'. But by that it means that
non-medical care should not be withheld from such a baby.
If, however, such a baby developed complications and it was
rejected by its parents, doctors would not be obliged to

intervene medically. But if handicapped infants have the same rights as other babies, why should they be deprived of the medical care that would be instantly forthcoming if a normal infant got into difficulties?

Surely the crucial factor is the intention and we must ask what is the intention of doctors who do not prescribe active treatment for some handicapped children. Their intention is, out of the highest motives, to cause the patient's death. As John Harris has argued: 'Selective treatment of severely handicapped children is calculated to result in their deaths. . . . It may seem tendentious to talk of patients "marked for death", but non-treatment is a death-dealing device.' There have been suggestions that the law should be amended to cover such cases. Diana and Malcolm Brahams, for example, have presented a draft Bill on the treatment of chronically disabled infants which is said to have been informally commended by the Director of Public Prosecutions. But it is probably impossible to construct a law that will cover all clinical eventualities and not restrict a doctor's freedom to treat his patient in the patient's best interests. The problem is that, in the current vacuum, doctors' value judgements may be unacceptably disparate and may even conflict with the view of society at large about what is morally right. The law may be too blunt an instrument—although it should always be available, as in the Alexandra case, as a last resort—but this does not mean that some more finely tuned device is not urgently needed.

Abortion

The change in the abortion law, with the passing of the Abortion Act 1967, was a watershed in medical thinking. As Mason and McCall Smith have commented: 'The moment the Act was accepted by doctors was the moment the profession abrogated a main tenet of its Hippocratic conscience—as late as 1968, the Declaration of Geneva, as amended in Sydney, was reiterating "I will maintain the utmost respect for human life from the time of conception".' By 1970, the Declaration of Oslo, while retaining this moral principle, had changed the tune: 'Diversity of response to this situation (the conflict of vital interests of the mother with vital interests of the child) results from the diversity of attitudes towards the life of the unborn child. This is a matter of individual conviction and conscience. . . .'

For the first time, modern medicine flirted with the concept of the wanted and the unwanted. This profound change in the law came about as a result of an equally profound change in society's attitudes. The overriding reason for the change was a utilitarian one—that the rate of maternal death and damage from back-street, illegal abortions was unacceptable as was the hypocrisy and inequality of the situation in which the rich had access to relatively safe abortions while the poor did not. There was also anxiety about the value of the lives of damaged or unwanted children, as well as concern about over-population and an acknowledgement of the decline in traditional religious beliefs. It was a good example of the way in which medical ethics adapt and change to meet the changing requirements of a society. For those with absolute views there is no problem. For Roman Catholics, for example, abortion can never be permitted because since a human person with its immortal soul is formed at conception, any destruction of that conceptus is murder. A parallel, if antithetical, certainty characterises those who believe that a woman has an absolute right over her own body, and since a foetus is merely a part of that body, it is a woman's right to choose whether a pregnancy should continue or be terminated.

The attitude embodied by the law, and accepted by the majority of doctors, falls between these two extreme positions. It does not place an absolute value upon human life so that a foetus has to be saved at all costs. But it places a very high value upon human life, so that any destruction of the foetus has to be capable of justification. It is a principle which has been dubbed by at least one commentator 'justifiable foeticide'. It is not considered justifiable to abort a foetus for social convenience, for example because the birth coincides with a planned holiday, but only if the birth presents a threat to the physical or mental health of the mother, or if there is a risk that the child, if born, will suffer serious physical or mental handicap. This appears to reflect the way in which doctors have traditionally approached the inherent contradiction in their ethical teaching, between the need to preserve life and the need to relieve suffering; there is no ethical duty to preserve life at all costs if the price of that life is the cause or prolongation of suffering.

The problem, however, is one of definition and boundaries. For a start, how is one to define or measure suffering? Pregnant women are now regularly screened to determine whether the child will be born affected by spina bifida. Given the likelihood of suffering among infants born with this tragic condition, it seems entirely reasonable for women to be offered abortions in such circumstances. It is also consistent with the value judgements made after birth, since most doctors would withhold treatment, with the consequences we have described, from the most damaged spina bifida babies on the grounds that the quality of their lives would be too poor. (It is hard, incidentally, to present a convincing argument as to why it is permissible to destroy such a life inside the uterus but it is nevertheless morally wrong to destroy it after it has been born.)

But what about situations in which trophoblastic screening establishes no more than the likelihood of handicap? Should an abortion be performed in such circumstances, where there is a possibility that the child will actually be normal? What if screening becomes so precise that it can determine that, say, rubella damage in a particular foetus has only affected the hearing, but the rest of the foetus is developing normally? How serious a handicap does there have to be to justify a therapeutic abortion? And what about the diagnosis of Down's Syndrome in the foetus as a result of amniocentesis? At present, diagnosis of such a handicap during pregnancy means that the mother is offered an abortion. But as we have said already, such a child may well live a reasonable life for many years. So on what basis is the abortion justified? It may be argued that there is no way of knowing how bad the handicap is; or that the birth of such a child would damage the mother's mental health. But even if these arguments applied, is there not a glaring inconsistency in attitudes which permit the abortion of Down's babies without a murmur, yet—at least in some sections of the population—object to such children being deprived of an equal right to life after they are born?

Another source of problems for doctors is the so-called 'social' reason for an abortion. This is because environmental or social reasons may be taken into account when deciding on the risk to the mother's health. The Lane committee on the Abortion Act, while reaffirming that Parliament's intention as enacted was to permit abortion only on medical grounds, conceded nevertheless that '. . . the subsection is regarded by many people within, as well as outside, the medical profession as meaning that an undesirable environmental situation of the mother of itself suffices to justify abortion'.

The concern has arisen because society in general does not think that social reasons are sufficient justification for destroying partly formed human life. Supporters of the attitude that a woman has an absolute right to choose, however, disagree since they say that the mother's rights are absolute. It is doubtful, however, whether this attitude would stand up to rigorous scrutiny. As Roger Wertheimer has pointed out:

Few liberals really regard abortion, at least in the later stages, as a bit of elective surgery. Suppose a woman had her fifth-month foetus aborted purely out of curiosity as to what it looked like, and perhaps then had it bronzed. Who among us would not deem both her and her actions reprehensible? Or, to go from the lurid to the ridiculous, suppose a wealthy woman, a Wagner addict, got an abortion in her fourth month because she suddenly realised that she would come to term during the Bayreuth festival. Only an exceptional liberal would not blanch at such behaviour.

The point is that, while we may say that there are circumstances in which the foetus's life can be ended, we have sufficient regard for its claim to life to say that such actions have to be justifiable. Curiosity to see what it would look like cast in bronze, or a desire not to miss the Bayreuth festival, would not meet those criteria. The difficulty lies in deciding what would. As Alastair Campbell, a lecturer in Christian ethics, has written:

In the majority of cases, the doctor will be presented with a complex set of psychological and social variables for assessment. Unless he takes a strictly 'medical' interpretation of 'risk to health' and accepts applications only from the physically ill or from people with a clearly diagnosed psychiatric disorder, he will be left with the problem of deciding how to assess the 'risks' to his patient . . . Obviously there may be straightforward economic factors to assess, but these again will often have to be seen in the context of the predicted attitudes to the new baby of the parent or parents. Perhaps most difficult of all to decide is the degree of disruption of the present life style or future plans of the pregnant woman which can or should be tolerated. For example, are disruption of an academic career, the necessity to give up a job or the anticipated social disgrace of an illegitimate birth undue risks to mental health?

A final consideration is the future well-being of the foetus if it is born into a situation in which the mother cannot, or will not, care for it. If a child is 'unwanted', is it better to prevent it from developing human awareness rather than subject it to the pain of rejection or the potential emotional insecurity of adoption?

In vitro fertilisation

The technique of *in vitro* fertilisation, where an ovum is fertilised by a sperm outside the body and then replaced in the uterus, has already transformed the lives of many otherwise childless couples, and no doubt its beneficial effects will multiply as the technique is improved and perfected. But more than perhaps any other single medical scientific advance, it has opened up a veritable Pandora's box of ethical dilemmas. Most of these are discussed elsewhere in this book, but there is a particular problem associated with the technique which can only be solved if we agree on the point at which life begins and the value that we place on it. This is the problem of what should be done with the spare embryos developed by IVF but not implanted in the womb. This problem was given a further dimension by the revelation that some of these embryos were being used for research. Dr Robert Edwards, who pioneered the technique with Mr Patrick Steptoe, was reported as saying that such research had helped him perfect the technique of growing embryos outside the womb, and he believed it would help him vastly improve the fertilisation rate of success. He also argued that such research could help us understand the cause of Down's Syndrome, to ensure that embryos reimplanted in the womb are genetically normal and to find out why some foetuses are rejected. Dr Edwards was not alone in this field. *New Scientist* reported that researchers at the Medical Research Council's Unit of Reproductive Biology in Edinburgh had grown ova to the blastocyst or eight-cell stage from women who had consented to sterilisation.

They then killed and fixed the embryos in order to look for chromosomal defects (as part of the test-tube programme). John Bancroft, the acting head of the unit, said that whether or not to do such research is 'not a simple ethical decision'. He said that researchers 'have to get into it, before deciding the real issues. These are just too difficult to decide in advance.' At this stage, he said, such research is reasonable, especially if it is associated with in vitro fertilisation. He added that human life, unless it leads to human existence, 'is not much'.

If one believes that life exists from the one-cell stage, then there can be no doubt that the IVF embryo is a form of life, just as a one-cell embryo is a form of very primitive life inside the uterus. The question then is, how much protection should we give that embryo? There is no question that the research will benefit it, since by definition it is killed to enable the research to take place. But if such research benefits humanity in general, shouldn't it be allowed to take place? Of course, as we show in our discussion of research ethics, research on the living should not take place without their informed consent. But we cannot escape the fact that an embryo of a few days gestation does not have the same rights as a human being after birth. Indeed, one might say that if we destroy embryos within the womb, as we do in abortion, why should we be particularly concerned about killing them in a petri-dish? It could be argued that abortions are only performed for therapeutic purposes, but then again such therapeutic purposes may bear no relation to the interests of the foetus; its rights are submerged by the rights of the mother. So why should we object if the rights of the IVF foetus are submerged by the rights of, say, future generations of children who might be saved from the Down's Syndrome that would otherwise have afflicted them?

Clifford Grobstein, professor of biological science and public policy at the University of California, has recognised that medical ethics, and indeed the ethics of society at large, are unable at present to cope with this problem.

The embryo doesn't necessarily deserve protection until it has some sense of emotional identification with another human being, and an inner life, some self-awareness. . . . It is probably never appropriate to treat a developing human being as experimental tissue; on the other hand, we shouldn't treat it as a fully developed human being. We have to consider all the traditions that led people to protect the helpless and have to come up with an acceptable solution.

However, achieving a consensus on this is far from easy. Quite apart from disagreements between people of different disciplines, opinions between doctors appear to be deeply divided. For example, in its evidence to the government inquiry into human fertilisation and embryology, the Royal College of General Practitioners wrote:

Although there are conflicting views about the onset of human life, the process can be considered to commence at fertilisation, since this is the point at which a genetically complete embryo is formed. From that moment, therefore, the embryo should be treated with respect, and experimentation on human embryos should be subject to the same ethical considerations as on children and adults. Experimentation on embryos has been going on for some time. Advances in medical science were made through unethical experiments such as those performed on human subjects during the last world war. However beneficial the information gained, the continuation of such unethical experiments cannot be justified.

On the other hand, the ethics committee of the Royal College of Obstetricians and Gynaecologists has written:

the fact that the embryo is genetically coded to become an adult human being does not ipso facto prohibit its use as a subject for biomedical research. Human reason and conscience have to determine when it would be wrong to carry out such research. The judgment must relate to its growth, especially its neural development, and codes of practice should be framed accordingly.

Edwards believes that spare embryos could be used to improve techniques of overcoming infertility. He also considers that it would be possible to take cells from early embryos to help existing children, in the form of bone-marrow transplants for example. In this he maintains that the claim to life of the 14-day embryo should be subservient to the interests of the child which has been born. Others believe that the time is not far off when it would be possible so to manipulate the genes of the pre-implantation embryo as to prevent the development of such conditions as cystic fibrosis in the resulting baby. In these matters, the RCOG ethics committee supports the published views of the Medical Research Council that 'scientifically sound research on the processes and products of *in vitro* fertilisation between human gametes is ethically acceptable and should be allowed to proceed on condition both that there is no intention to transfer to the uterus any embryo resulting from or used in such experiments and also that the aim of the research is clearly defined and directly relevant to clinical problems such as contraception or the differential diagnosis and treatment of infertility and inherited diseases. Human embryos employed in this way should not be allowed to develop beyond the stage of early neural development . . . and such research should be subject to informed consent of the donor or donors.'

The conflict between the two colleges' views may be caused by a brand new scientific conundrum, but the essentials of the conflict are nevertheless the familiar contradictory principles of utilitarianism and autonomy. The RCOG, with suitable safeguards, has decided that the beneficial results of such research outweigh any rights the embryo may possess; the RCGP maintains that the autonomy of the embryo is the most important consideration.

Euthanasia

Literally, euthanasia means a gentle and easy death, but the subject is usually subdivided into passive and active euthanasia. Passive euthanasia involves doing nothing to actively kill a patient but allowing him to die by failing to take steps to prolong his life. This, as we saw earlier in this chapter, is acceptable to many doctors, although there are considerable problems about deciding on the values that should govern such a decision. However, the great majority of doctors draw a firm distinction between passive and active euthanasia, in which the doctor would take active steps to kill the patient. The BMA has campaigned vigorously against several Parliamentary Bills that have sought to legalise voluntary, active euthanasia.

Voluntary euthanasia describes a situation in which the patient asks to die; involuntary euthanasia one in which the patient could ask to die, but does not, and is killed nevertheless. There are also circumstances where the patient cannot make such a decision at all, because he is comatose or senile, for example, or is a newborn baby.

Involuntary euthanasia is wrong, since it involves ignoring a person's autonomous rights and killing him; it is therefore indistinguishable from murder. So the controversy centres around the questions of whether there is any moral difference between passive and active euthanasia, and if there is not, whether doctors should apply it, and if so, whether it should be applied both to patients who ask for it and those who cannot formulate or express a wish.

We should not lightly dismiss the reasons why someone wants a doctor to help him to die. He may be in great pain from a terminal illness—although, as the hospice movement has demonstrated, it should be possible for such pain to be alleviated with proper medical and nursing care, in which case the patient may cease to fret for an early death. But there may be cases where attention to bodily needs cannot alter the sound judgement of a person that he would be better off dead. For example, a young person paralysed from the neck down may take a calm and rational decision that there is nothing about his life that he values and moreover he wants to end the misery that his handicap causes to his family. If he approaches his doctor to put an end to his life, is not the doctor wrong to override the autonomy of that young person who has a right to decide whether he lives or dies?

It is certainly true that we allow that young person the right to take his own life, to commit suicide, if he wishes. It remains a crime, however, to aid or abet that suicide. Consequently it is illegal if not unethical for a doctor to assist in that process. In refusing to do so, the doctor is not denying that person's autonomy—he can throw himself off a cliff in his wheel-chair, if he wishes—but he is refusing to become its tool. If he were to agree, he would turn himself into an executioner.

But, it might be argued, that same doctor might go straight from that young person to an old man suffering from senile dementia and pneumonia and he may decide not to give him antibiotics since it is kinder to let him die. Isn't that the same? The intention of the doctor is that the old man should die and it is crucially important that the doctor should take responsibility for both his actions and his inactions. But it is still important for a doctor not to be seen as an executioner, both from the point of view of his own self-image and for his relationship with his patients. Moreover, it would be hard to be certain all the time about the patient's true intentions when he made his request for euthanasia, or that he might not have changed his mind.

Unless a participant in the debate wishes to give different rights to different individuals, there are no new arguments to be deployed. Euthanasia is a euphemism for 'killing or letting die' from an earlier part of this century. On strictly moral grounds, the distinction between killing and allowing to die is, as we have said, hard to sustain. But this does not necessarily mean that we should follow the argument to one role and license doctors to kill. There are powerful arguments against this. As for active euthanasia done to people who cannot give consent, Jonathan Glover points out that: 'The question is: given the case which exists in some circumstances for deliberately terminating life where the person is not in a position to request it, can we act on this without contributing towards attitudes of indifference or worse towards killing in less justifiable situations?'

There is another question which must be asked after that. Given that we already allow life to be terminated which we might otherwise save, because we feel that this is in the person's best interests, have we not already diluted our repugnance at causing death and have we not fatally weakened our defences against unjustifiable indifference or worse?

3
RESEARCH AND
EXPERIMENTATION

In the middle part of the nineteenth century, seminal papers by scientists like Francis Galton led to a generally agreed form of attack on problems in science—the scientific method. The hypothetico–deductive approach embodied in the 'scientific method' was an important new tool in the *armamentarium* of scientists. Bertrand Russell describes the impact of science on public opinion in *Power* in the following terms:

It is customary nowadays (1938) to decry Reason as a force in human affairs, yet the rise of science is an overwhelming argument on the other side. The men of science proved to intelligent laymen that a certain kind of intellectual outlook ministers to military prowess and wealth; these ends were so ardently desired that the new intellectual outlook overcame that of the Middle Ages, in spite of the force of tradition and the revenues of the Church and the sentiments associated with Catholic theology. The world ceased to believe that Joshua caused the sun to stand still, because Copernican astronomy was useful in navigation; it abandoned Aristotle's physics, because Galileo's theory of falling bodies made it possible to calculate the trajectory of a cannon-ball; it rejected the story of the flood, because geology is useful in mining and so on. . . . From this example, something may be learnt as to the power of Reason in general. In the case of science, Reason prevailed over prejudice because it provided means of realising existing purposes, and because the proof that it did so was overwhelming. Those who maintain that Reason has no power in human affairs overlook these two conditions. If, in the name of Reason, you summon a man to alter his fundamental purposes—to pursue, say, the general happiness rather than his own power—you will fail, and you will deserve to fail, since Reason alone cannot determine the ends of life. And you will fail equally if you attack deep-seated prejudices while your argument is open to question, or is so difficult that only men of science can see its force. But if you can prove, by evidence that is

56

convincing to every sane man who takes the trouble to examine it, that you possess the means of facilitating existing desires, you may hope, with a certain degree of confidence, that men will ultimately believe what you say.

In the twentieth century, medical research has been held to be necessary to benefit mankind, and the subjects were reasonably content. Remember that during the First World War, more babies died each week during the perinatal period than there were soldiers killed in the trenches. This perinatal mortality has been sharply reduced, largely as the result of careful research leading to changes in social policy.

But times have changed. The watershed was undoubtedly the discovery of the 'medical' experiments conducted by the Nazis. At the Nuremberg tribunal, Brigadier General Telford Taylor stated that the 23 Nazi doctors on trial had received human subjects in wholesale lots—'200 Jews . . . , 50 gypsies, 500 tubercular Poles, or 1,000 Russians' for experiments which 'revealed nothing which civilised medicine can use'. We have mentioned the nature of these experiments elsewhere, and make the point that they were not 'medical' at all, but designed to further the cause of the master-race rather than to benefit humanity, to inflict bestial suffering and death rather than to discover new ways of healing the sick or preserving life. Nevertheless, they were medical experiments in that they were carried out by doctors, using scientific methods of analysis in however warped a cause. Thus, after the Nuremberg trials, there evolved a code of practice to ensure that medicine could not be perverted in this way again. The Nuremberg Code consisted of ten points, of which the first read:' The voluntary consent of the subject is absolutely essential. . . .' The principles embodied in this code were refined in the Declaration of Helsinki in 1964, which laid down the difference betwen therapeutic experiments, in which clinical research is combined with professional care, and non-therapeutic research, in which experiments are not supposed to benefit the subject but are purely scientific.

Since the war, however, medical research has generated a multitude of developments which have outstripped our codes

of morality. We can transplant hearts, kidneys, livers—
before long, maybe the brain itself. We can screen patients
for more and more varieties of genetic damage, inching ever
closer to the genetically engineered perfect human race.

In addition, the old paternalistic certainties have disappeared. Patients are no longer prepared to accept unques-
tioningly what their doctors tell them. Society now places
greater value upon individual autonomy, the patient's ability
or claim to decide what should or should not happen to his or
her body. The trouble is that medical experiments on human
subjects must entail some erosion of each subject's right to
self-determination. The Declaration of Geneva says, after all,
'The health of my patient shall be my first consideration'. If
this were taken literally and interpreted rigidly, no medical
experiments upon human beings could be permitted at all.
Yet since such experiments are necessary for the progress of
medicine and thus for the benefit of humanity, a balance
must be found. It is a matter of weighing risks against
benefits. The Declaration of Helsinki says that biomedical
research involving human subjects cannot legitimately be
carried out unless the importance of the objective is in
proportion to the inherent risk to the subject. Every such
research project, it says, should be preceded by a careful
assessment of the predictable risks in comparison with the
foreseeable benefits.

Concern for the interests of the subjects, says the Declaration of Helsinki, must always prevail over the interests of
science and society. But taken literally, this would mean that
very little research on human subjects was possible since
virtually every medical procedure involves some degree of
risk. How are the risks and benefits to be weighed? The
American ethicist, Hans Jonas, wrote a classic article in 1969,
'Philosophical reflections on experimenting with human
subjects', in which he tried to resolve the dilemma.

Jonas started by placing such emphasis on the interests of
the research subjects that research on humans could not be
justified except in cases of emergency. The improvement of
society was not a sufficient justification to ask people to
accept risks or burdens. Yet by the end of his article, Jonas
had managed to argue himself into exactly the opposite

corner. For as he acknowledged, if medical science were to make any progress at all, experimentation on people had to take place. So he ended by arguing for the safeguard that no experiments on patients should take place if they were unrelated to their disease. So he came down after all on the utilitarian side.

This apparently oscillatory argument illustrates the deficiencies of the absolutists' case, as well as providing a warning against rampant utilitarianism. Human experimentation is an area where there are ethical arguments against both action and inaction. How can there be an absolute moral answer? In an article in the *Journal of Medical Ethics*, Arthur Schafer of Manitoba University's Department of Philosophy put the case for both sides: 'The ideals of distributive justice and individual dignity should be used as a "brake" or check against the sort of crass benefit-producing ethic which would classify some individuals as fit to be conscripted forcibly for some social end because they are burdensome and therefore socially "expendable". But then he went on to say that it may be that the benefits of research are so great that we have no alternative but to use human subjects.

After all, human dignity can be severely undermined by serious illness as well as by the human experimentation designed to eliminate such illness. There is an ethical cost attaching to not doing such research as well as to proceeding with it. If one is faced with a choice between protecting personal dignity by imposing a total ban on experimentation or, alternatively, protecting the dignity of potential beneficiaries of research (of present and future generations) by permitting such experimentation to proceed, it is defensible to be influenced by the numbers of people affected and the degree of benefit and harm to both.

This is the middle ground of the Helsinki Declaration. It is not just a morally permissible position to hold—it appears to be the only possible position to hold since both the alternative extremes are unacceptable. But there is a further dimension to this problem. Behind Hans Jonas's conclusions, behind the Helsinki Declaration itself is the tacit assumption that experimentation, whether on humans or otherwise, always produces a benign result—that medical progress, the advancement of medical science, inevitably equates with a benefit to mankind. But the modern dilemma is that some of these advances turn out to be two-edged swords. Heart transplants, for example, can provide a few heart-disease sufferers with otherwise unattainable years of healthy life. But unless such experimental surgery is controlled, the cost of the research distorts health funding so that many other people suffering from more easily treatable complaints cannot be helped. Additionally, the numbers who do survive for long periods are extremely small at present. Yet to suggest that such research should be restricted creates a furore, at least partly because the proponents of the argument say that further research will improve the techniques and drugs making the benefits available to larger numbers of people and reducing costs.

Take the dramatic improvements in perinatal care. We can now save many more defective newborn babies who previously would have died. Yet by saving them, we are preserving lives that are often handicapped, sometimes extremely so. Presumably, the earlier we are able to save sick newborn infants, the greater the likelihood of preserving life that is chronically impaired. Is that really a development that is of unmitigated benefit to humanity?

At the same time, our capacity to screen pregnant women for genetic damage to their unborn babies proceeds apace, with the underlying assumption that such genetic damage legitimises an abortion. But where do we draw the line at the kind of genetic damage that does not qualify for an abortion? And how do we square the assumption behind such screening, that imperfect human beings should not be born, with the impulse at the other end of the nine-month process, to save newborn babies, however defective?

In other words, the question has to be asked whether anyone has an absolute right to seek medical knowledge for its own sake, which will produce tension with the rights of the research subject, and other people in the community who may be affected by the financial consequences of the outcome of the research. Alternatively we may ask whether medical research should take its place as part of a planned social philosophy. As Pellegrino and Thomasma wrote, 'a philosopy of medicine is needed to help clarify medicine's goals in relationship to those of a technological civilisation. Medicine suffers from an abundance of means and a poverty of ends.'

Consent

At the heart of the Declaration of Helsinki lies the emphasis on the informed consent of the research subject to experimentation. This is, on the face of it, the most powerful safeguard that can be devised against exploitation. It protects the individual's rights over his or her own body, and respects the important principle of personal autonomy; it provides a safety catch to ensure that the value of an individual life does not get thrown overboard in the quest for utilitarian goals. But, that said, it is a safeguard that is fraught with difficulties. The Declaration of Helsinki states:

In any research on human beings, each potential subject must be adequately informed of the aims, methods, anticipated benefits and potential hazards of the study and the discomfort it may entail. He or she should be informed that he or she is at liberty to abstain from participation in the study and that he or she is free to withdraw his or her consent to participation at any time. The doctor should then obtain the subject's freely-given informed consent, preferably in writing.

This in itself, however, is a difficult criterion to fulfil. What, for example, is 'adequately informed'? Many have criticised this term as being so vague as to be positively unhelpful. As Mr Justice Kirby, the former chairman of the Australian Law Reform Commission commented:

It must be frankly recognised that to some extent at least the notion of 'informed consent' is simply an ideal to which daily practice can only aim. Some commentators have suggested that it is an ideal in the nature of a myth. This is said because it is impossible for the health care professional to impart to the patient every facet of his knowledge and expertise involved in this decision. A lifetime or at least many years of experience and judgement may lie behind the decision. This cannot be imparted, in the real world, in the space of a 30-minute consultation. Patients vary enormously both in their interest in and capacity to absorb information about medical procedures. It is the very expertise of the health care professional that brought the patient to him. To this extent consent is 'that by a less knowledgeable person to one who is more knowledgeable'.

Kirby then went on to refer to research which proved the inadequacies of so-called informed consent:

Within one day of signing forms for chemotherapy, radiation therapy or surgery, 220 cancer patients completed a test of their recall of the material in the consent explanation and filled out a questionnaire regarding their opinions of its purpose, content and implications. Only 60% understood the purpose and nature of the procedure, and only 55% correctly listed every major risk of complication. We found that three factors were related to inadequate recall: education, medical status and the care with which patients thought they had read their consent forms before signing. Only 40% of the patients had read the form 'carefully'. Most believed that consent forms were meant to 'protect the physician's rights'.

If, however, we said that because informed consent is an unattainable goal human research is unethical, experimentation would grind to a halt and so would the advance of medical science. Some might say that since this must remain an academic exercise, we should wash our hands of the issue of informed consent completely and leave it to the doctors to regulate themselves. But, as Kirby comments, this won't do.

The days of paternalistic medicine are numbered. The days of unquestioning trust of the patient also appear to be numbered. The days of complete and general consent to anything a doctor cared to do appear numbered. Nowadays doctors, out of respect for themselves and for their patients (to say nothing for deference to the law) must increasingly face the obligation of securing informed consent from the patient for the kind of therapeutic treatment proposed.

There is no completely satisfactory formula, he suggests, for informed consent, but what the doctor can do, at the very least, is to remember that the moral principle behind informed consent is respect for the integrity and autonomy of the patient. But this is not the only problem with informed consent. For the Declaration of Helsinki contained a major *caveat* to this requirement on which it lays such stress. When medical research is combined with professional care, it says: 'If the doctor considers it essential not to obtain informed consent, the specific reasons for this proposal should be stated in the experimental protocol for transmission to the independent committees.'

So, having laboured consent, the Declaration somewhat surprisingly then permits exceptions to this golden rule. Presumably, its drafters had in mind precisely the kind of case that occurred in Britain in 1981 and caused considerable controversy. In that case, a widow of 84 died from bone-marrow depression induced by fluorouracil during a controlled clinical trial. She had been included in the trial although her consent had not been obtained. The woman was one of several patients suffering from cancer of the colon or rectum who were divided into three groups, each being given different treatments. The local ethical committees apparently decided that seeking informed consent from each patient was not appropriate. At the inquest into the woman's death, the coroner suggested that the whole idea of concealed controlled trials should be brought to public notice for proper discussion. *The Lancet* was outraged and wrote a strong leader condemning what had happened.

The fluorouracil trial, involving a portal catheter and a toxic drug, should—on the criteria of both variance from standard procedure and degree of risk—have had special consent. . . . If the patient is not capable of understanding the basic plan of mangement, he or she should not be included in the trial. No-one pretends that these matters are easy for doctor or patient, but it is important that the clinical research exercise remains a partnership built on trust.

To which the chairman of one of the research ethical committees involved, Owen Lyndon Wade of the Queen Elizabeth Hospital, Birmingham, wrote an equally outraged reply. It was understood that all the patients would have to consent to a major operation, and it was the committee's opinion that the injection of drugs into the portal vein was part of the surgical operation, a procedure used since 1970. He went on:

Fully informed consent for the comparison of the two drugs used in this trial could only be obtained by explaining to the patients why the drugs were being given and how unfavourable the prognosis after operation was going to be. We thought this would be an unacceptable psychological trauma for many of the patients who had just agreed to a major operation for cancer. . . . The trial protocol does not stop surgeons obtaining fully informed consent about the use of drugs but it does not make it mandatory. We agreed with the protocol because we felt that the quality of the limited post-operative life of many of these patients would be impaired if, in explaining the trial, the grim prognosis was revealed.

This answer rather begged the wider question of truth-telling to terminally ill patients. While no one would suggest that the grim truth be broken to such patients with brutal speed, nevertheless the implication that these patients were going to remain ignorant of their extremely limited life-span is a little disconcerting. But whatever the rights or wrongs of such ignorance, the argument fails to confront the central issue here—that it is wrong to experiment upon a dying patient without his or her consent. To do so upsets the delicate balance that must be struck between respect for an individual's life and concern for utilitarian goals. Yet the committee chairman was quite right to point out that this trial had been carried out in full accord with the Declaration of Helsinki. *The Lancet* fulminated that members of ethical committees should be better informed about the ethical codes drawn up by international bodies, but it was *The Lancet* which had apparently overlooked the *caveat* in the Declaration, that informed consent can be dispensed with in therapeutic trials.

Controlled clinical trials

The fundamental problem with controlled clinical trials in

which one kind of treatment is given to one group of patients and another kind to another group was expressed succinctly by Mason and McCall Smith. They wrote that even the best designed trial has its built-in moral problem.

Depending on how one looks at it, on the one hand a relatively untried treatment which may do harm is being given to one group, while on the other a treatment which may be of considerable benefit is being withheld from a similar group. The doctor is doing his best for patients but the problem is to know what is best; put another way, the ethical problem is not so much whether a patient will be completely cured by a new treatment but, rather, would he have improved faster if he had not been restrained by the experimental protocol.

The problem is actually immensely complicated because it involves a circular argument which goes like this. Randomised clinical trials can never be reconciled with the best treatment for the individual patient participating in those trials because of the element of random selection into experimental and control groups; but unless one conducts such a trial, one cannot know in advance what the best treatment for that particular patient actually is. D.W. Vere, of London Hospital's Department of Pharmacology and Therapeutics, put it like this:

First, it seems to me to be a matter of ineluctable logic that, if a group of colleagues agree that they would become convinced of a treatment's superiority for the group after, and only after, a prefixed level of statistical significance had been exceeded, then until that moment is reached the best treatment for every individual is either of the therapies under test, chosen at random. It would surely be unethical not to make a trial. Once the uncertainty has been removed it is unethical to make one. And notice that this has little to do with what those investigators may believe up to that point, what hunches they may have, or what their friends may say. Until the facts have been demonstrated, whatever they may believe, they do not know. Their level of foundation for their beliefs must be raised by evidence to the point where no reasonable person is likely to reject it. Until that point, the best therapy for the individual is the random choice.

That is all very well when the arguments against two alternative therapies are finely balanced—for example, if two centres are using different treatments and the relative superiority of either of them can only be determined by a controlled trial. And it is certainly true that no patient should participate in such a trial if the proposed treatment is thought to be second best; the Declaration of Helsinki states that every patient in a study, including those in the control group, should be assured of the best proven therapeutic and diagnostic method. But what if there is more than a hunch but less than certainty about a particular treatment option? An example of such a dilemma was presented in 1982 when, after much dithering, the Medical Research Council finally decided to go ahead with its plan to establish once and for all whether vitamin supplements prevented spina bifida in babies. This decision caused intense controversy, with several medical teams refusing to take part. This was because research that had been running for six years or so, under Professor Richard Smithells at Leeds University, had already indicated persuasively that supplements of multivitamins and folic acid prevented spina bifida.

But Professor Smithells' research was not conclusive; to be absolutely certain, there had to be a control group of women who would not be given vitamin supplements—women who ran a higher than average risk of carrying a spina bifida baby. If one followed Vere's logic—and the MRC, by its decision, seemed to be doing just that—the trial was necessary because otherwise no one could know whether the supplements were necessary or not. But Vere would consequently have to accept that such a trial might well result in a number of spina bifida babies being born who otherwise might have been born healthy. Complaining that this would only be with the benefit of hindsight in this particular case would not do, because there were grounds for believing, before the trial started, that such supplements did have this beneficial effect.

The Declaration of Helsinki draws a crucial distinction between therapeutic trials—that is, experiments that combine medical research with professional care—and non-therapeutic research. The former must, by definition, involve patients. The latter, it says, should involve volunteers—although it then states that these might be either healthy people or patients, as long as the experiments are not related to the patients' own illnesses. This seems rather to undermine the important distinction between the two types of experiment, since any patient is vulnerable and under stress. But that apart, the distinction is held to be a vital one. Thurstan Brewin, of the Institute of Radiotherapeutics and Oncology at Glasgow's Belvedere Hospital, has said that this fundamental distinction is too often missed and leads to confusion about the aims and ethics of randomised trials. It was not true, he said, that patients in such trials were merely being used for the benefit of others. Controlled trials were conducted with the sole aim of benefiting the patient. There was no such thing as a single best treatment for every situation. Doctors had to choose from several best treatments, themselves a balance between hazard and benefit. In a trial, this choice was made by random selection, but with the aim of finding the best treatment for the patient. He wrote: 'A doctor who contributes to randomised treatment trials should not be thought of as a research worker, but simply as a clinician with an ethical duty to his patients not to go on giving them treatments without doing anything possible to assess their true worth.' But this, surely, is to miss the point of the controversy. Whatever the Declaration of Helsinki says, the distinction between therapeutic and non-therapeutic trials is by no means clear-cut. There is a distinct grey area in which research done for the benefit of the patient is not done solely for that purpose but to benefit future patients as well. The second element inescapably undermines the moral integrity of the former. Hence the problem.

But surely the essential safeguard for the patient in such a delicate matter is the patient's informed consent to such experiments. Especially in cases of serious illness, it seems obvious that different varieties of treatment should be tried out—but it also seems obvious that this should only be done with the patient's consent. This is the vital point that was ignored in the case of the woman who died from the results of the fluorouracil trial. But Thurstan Brewin disagreed. He wrote that because randomised treatment was not 'research' but an honest attempt to find the best treatment for an individual patient, consent could be dispensed with. To justify this position, he said:

Randomisation is bound to sound strange and wrong to many patients. If there are doctors and lawyers who see it only as 'human experimentation', what chance is there for the majority of patients grasping the need for it and the ethics of it? The mere fact that special written consent is thought to be necessary may give the patient (and his relatives and everyone else) the wrong impression. Secondly, if informed consent is to come anywhere near to being what it is supposed to be, we have to describe not only likely hazards but unlikely ones—and we have to do this not just for one treatment policy but for those in the randomised trial and others not in the trial. Increasing detail often leads to increasing confusion—for example, as to which hazard goes with which treatment. If all this is written down for the patient, there may be less risk of certain kinds of misunderstanding, but cold print may still further increase the risk of exaggerated fears. Many patients . . . have no wish to hear about all the benefits and hazards of different options. They just want to get started with a line of treatment that is fully supported by their doctor—a doctor whom they trust (if they do not, they should choose another), who is sincerely interested in their problems, anxious to help and ethically totally committed to their care—all of which is fully consistent with giving randomised treatment, with or without special consent.

Is it? Thurstan Brewin's argument seems highly tendentious. If randomisation is not only proper but is the best course of action for a particular patient, it should be explained as such. To say there is not much chance of such a subtle argument being understood is no reason for doing away with the explanation altogether. It means, rather, that the principle should be explained better—and if the patient disagrees, and concludes that it is too much like human experimentation and that he or she does not wish to participate, then it is surely the patient's right to come to such a conclusion, ill-informed as Brewin thinks it may be, and refuse to take part. And to say that increasing detail leads to increasing confusion is again to beg the question of the patient's right to know. It is possible to explain even complicated issues without causing confusion—time-consuming and difficult maybe, but possible. To argue that detail equals confusion is an example of the worst kind of paternalism and an excuse for misleading a patient. Some patients undoubtedly do not want to be bothered with the risk/benefit equation of their treatment—but they should surely be given the chance at least to say whether they want to know or not. To move from saying that some patients don't want to know to saying that all patients should not be given the chance to know is a disturbing non sequitur. Truth-telling, essential throughout medicine, is an even more vital safeguard in the difficult area of experimentation. If patients don't want to be told, or can't give their informed consent for any reason, then they should not participate in the trial.

This dilemma was tackled by the Cancer Research Campaign working party in breast conservation. In November 1982 the Campaign launched a trial in early breast cancer designed to determine whether cutting out the tumour and giving radiotherapy, while conserving the breast, gave patients the same chance of survival and freedom from the disease as a mastectomy with radiotherapy. About 2,000 patients were needed for the trial, but the problem was that informed consent was believed to carry the risk of losing patients to the trial. Despite this risk, the working party came down firmly on the side of informed consent—but not without thinking through the disadvantages of this course of action.

Not unnaturally, a compassionate clinician is concerned that by so taking a patient into his confidence and declaring his own uncertainties, this will undermine his patient's trust in him and thus adversely affect the outcome of treatment. Are these fears justified? To some extent, they can be tested only by experience, but evidence suggests that uninformed patients may also be alarmed, anxious and subject to considerable stress precisely because they are being kept in the dark. They may privately suspect that bad news is being kept from them. Patients who genuinely do not want to know about their condition may say so frankly, in which case the doctor is relieved of the obligation to make other disclosures. A perceptive doctor will appreciate his patient's insecurities and be concerned to do all he can to improve her understanding of the situation. He should, however, also be aware that sometimes the patient who says: 'I leave it to you, doctor, you know best' may be expressing not so much genuine consent as an anxious wish to be compliant and cause as little trouble as possible.

However, the working party came to the conclusion that, despite the ambiguities of the Declaration of Helsinki, informed consent was essential. And unless doctors grasped the nettle of informed consent, warned the researchers, the results could be disastrous for society.

As a result of our deliberations, we have decided that it is now vitally important for the medical profession to brace itself to confront the issue of informed consent squarely, and to examine all its implications with the aim of hammering out an acceptable working ethic for future practice. If doctors, medical researchers and ethical committees are not prepared to collaborate in a joint initiative of this nature, it is all too probable that they will be overtaken by events in the undesirable and potentially extremely damaging shape of a public outcry. Should this happen, emotive and misinformed arguments will inevitably muddy the debate, polarise attitudes and force the profession into a defensive stance. It then risks being shown as confused and divided on a serious ethical issue which could cause it to suffer a dangerous loss of credibility as well as hampering the prospects for all future clinical trials.

The outcome of the researchers' discussions on this issue, and a measure of their concern, was a set of practical proposals for improving consent procedures. These involved:

1 giving eligible patients the option to take time to consider giving their consent;
2 making the consent form fairly non-specific but backed up by as much verbal explanation as possible;
3 obtaining the help of a trained nurse counsellor or some other suitably qualified person to obtain the consent;
4 making informed consent a top priority for an ethical committee's consideration of a particular trial;
5 emphasising the obligation upon doctors treating cancer patients who are not involved in clinical trials to discuss

alternative forms of treatment with those patients, even though they are not formally randomised.

Unless such a code is formulated quickly, said the researchers, patients and doctors will be scared off controlled trials and we shall be plunged back into the 'dark ages where therapeutic innovations were judged by intuition and wishful thinking'.

Patients who cannot give 'informed consent'

The ethical problems of clinical research are greatly magnified when the proposed subjects are thought incapable of giving their informed consent to the experiment—for example, children, prisoners or mentally handicapped or ill people. The dilemma is caused by the necessity to protect the vulnerable from exploitation, set against the occasional necessity to carry out research using subjects from one of these groups. The question is further complicated by the difference between therapeutic and non-therapeutic research. It may help to consider these different examples of the problem separately.

Children
Most of the argument about the ethics of research on children centres on the rights and wrongs of non-therapeutic research. But it is far from clear whether non-therapeutic research on children is actually permissible under the terms of the Declaration of Helsinki. It is true that the Declaration specifically mentions the legally incompetent subject of research, saying that in such cases informed consent should be obtained from the legal guardian or responsible relative. But this provision is contained in the declaration of general principles. In the section governing non-therapeutic research, which the Declaration carefully distinguishes from therapeutic research, it states categorically that 'The subjects should be volunteers—either healthy persons or patients for whom the experimental design is not related to the person's illness'. It is hard to imagine that a 'volunteer' can be someone whose

consent is impossible to obtain. One could certainly say that the informed consent of a guardian is the nearest one can get to consent for procedures involving a child, but it is clearly only the best possible substitute, which might be necessary in the interests of the child but which will not do when the research is nothing to do with the child's best interests.

In any event, is non-therapeutic research ever justifiable on children? The British Paediatric Association proposed guidelines in 1980 which were based on these assumptions:

1 that research involving children is important for the benefit of all children and should be supported and encouraged and conducted in an ethical manner;
2 that research should never be done on children if the same investigation could be done on adults;
3 that research which involves a child and is of no benefit to that child is not necessarily either unethical or illegal;
4 that the degree of benefit resulting from research should be assessed in relation to the risk/benefit ratio.

The BPA guidelines go on to provide examples of the different types of risk that need to be balanced against the likely benefits—but these tend to illustrate the immense difficulty in reaching such a balance. For example, during an abdominal operation a renal biopsy might be taken for research purposes. The risk would be more than minimal, say the guidelines, and the benefit would have to be very large to justify it—for instance, if the research aimed to resolve the problem of rejection of transplanted kidneys. Such a benefit, though, would seem to us to be far too removed from the child in question to justify the risk.

Another example involves glucose tolerance tests on a diabetic child, to discover how to prevent blindness in such children. The guidelines say that the risk of discomfort or pain to that child would be more than minimal, but might nevertheless be justified by the potential benefit. Any medical procedure, however minor, carries a degree of risk, however minimal, and there is a strong case for saying that even a negligible risk arising from an experimental procedure is unjustifiable in the light of the child's inability to give consent.

This concern for a child who is vulnerable because of the unusual discrepancy in power between the patient and the doctor does not seem to apply to research which can be done using procedures which are part of the ordinary care of the child—for example, feeding, weighing, measuring and clinically necessary pathology tests. It is the introduction of additional risk and distress which is unacceptable. Clearly, a ban on non-therapeutic research on children would mean losing the benefits to society that such research might bring. But as in all such matters a balance has to be sought with the rights of the individual. We draw the line at non-therapeutic research on adults without informed consent, so why should we adopt less stringent safeguards where children are concerned?

It can be argued that informed consent is provided in such cases by the parent or guardian. But while this may be good enough for therapeutic research, without which the individual child may be worse off, it is not good enough for non-therapeutic research. Moreover, the idea that the parent will automatically decide in the best interests of the child is not tenable. As Mason and McCall Smith point out, in recent years the law has increasingly questioned the concept of parental rights over the child and substituted the doctrine of the child's own rights. The child's best interests may not necessarily be served by the parents' decision. An example of this, in a medical context, was provided by the case of Alexandra, which was described in the previous chapter. The parents didn't want a life-saving operation performed on her; the court took the view that the parents had not decided in the baby's best interests and that the operation should proceed.

Clearly, such examples are rare, and taking the right of decision away from the parents is such a serious step that it should only occur in the rarest of cases.

The vast majority of parents would no doubt make decisions about their children's best interests with which doctors and the courts would not disagree. But it is necessary, nevertheless, for the courts to act in the last resort to decide what is in the best interests of the child. An expert third party assessment is even more important when experimentation on a child is being considered. If a doctor thinks that the parents are not acting in the child's best interests—as happens, for example, in cases involving Jehovah's Witnesses—the doctor can ask the courts to overrule the parents. But in cases of proposed therapeutic research, the parents and the doctor may unconsciously collude to reach a decision which is not in the child's best interests and it is important that the research should be carefully scrutinised by the hospital's ethical committee.

Mentally handicapped people

Mentally handicapped people are even more vulnerable than children, since they tend to live in institutions and may not have families who want anything to do with them. It is therefore vitally important that the Helsinki distinction between therapeutic research, which may benefit such people, and non-therapeutic research is maintained;—yet as we have already said, that distinction is often blurred in practice. Research that brings no benefit to mentally handicapped people should surely never be carried out on them—unless it involves, as with children, some normal procedure such as feeding or experiments carrying no risk whatever of danger or unpleasantness to the person, such as colour discrimination or hearing tests.

Therapeutic research should surely only be carried out on people who are mentally handicapped with the informed consent of the parents or nearest relatives. The repugnance attached to exploiting such entirely helpless and vulnerable people expressed itself most poignantly in the controversy over the experiments at Willowbrook, a residential school for mentally handicapped children in New York. This research, which began in 1956, involved deliberately infecting children at the school with viral hepatitis. The medical staff claimed that because most children admitted to the school became infected with hepatitis, it was better for them to be infected deliberately and isolated in a special unit. If this were the reason for the experiment, it would have fallen within the category of therapeutic research and thus might have been justified under the Declaration of Helsinki, since the consent of the parents had been obtained. But it was subsequently claimed that the experiment was continued because the staff wanted to continue to study hepatitis, and new measures which might have given the children protection from the disease were not used. If that were true, then the experiment would have been a repugnant example of exploitation. But in any event, even if it was a therapeutic experiment, it is hard to escape the thought that deliberate infection with a disease would not have been contemplated on normal children.

Mentally ill people

Mentally ill people are also extremely vulnerable, but for slightly different reasons. Whereas the mentally handicapped person is incapable of informed consent, mentally ill people will be able to provide informed consent in the vast majority of cases, even if they are detained in a psychiatric hospital under the Mental Health Act—yet it may be assumed, simply by virtue of their circumstances, that they are unable to do this. Once again, there should be no question of non-therapeutic research, since although patients may be capable of rational agreement, the fact of their incarceration means that they can never truly be 'volunteers'. They are patients; and although the Declaration of Helsinki explicitly provides for patients being used in such experiments provided the research is not related to their illness, it is hard to imagine that psychiatric patients would be used for such unrelated research. And even if they were, they would still be vulnerable because of their position.

However, therapeutic research on mentally ill people also presents grave ethical problems. Should the consent of a detained patient be sought to such procedures? Is it likely to be valid? Even if obtained and valid, is it enough to sanction such experiments? The problem was illustrated by Larry Gostin, the former legal director of Mind, the mental health charity, in a paper on psychosurgery in the *Journal of Social Welfare Law*. Psychosurgery is one of the most controversial experimental procedures used on mentally ill people. The controversy arose from arguments about the usefulness of such surgery and its ill-effects, considering that it irrevocably affects the patient's personality and attempts to control aberrant behaviour. Gostin wrote that consent of the patient was important, in that it upheld the autonomy and individual dignity of the individual. But that consent was itself fraught with problems:

The decision of some patients may also be affected by their perception that failure to consent to prescribed treatment may lead, in the case of informal patients, to the use of compulsory powers and, in the case of patients already detained, to prolonged confinement. The use of psychosurgery on compulsorily detained patients presents particular difficulties. The possibility has to be considered that individuals in confinement may be inherently likely to accept irreversible or unestablished treatment which they would not choose were they in a freer position or better circumstances.

And as Gostin has written elsewhere, there will always be circumstances, by virtue of the patient's illness, where consent is impossible to obtain but where such procedures as psychosurgery or electro-convulsive therapy may be necessary. The only safeguard, he concluded, was an independent multidisciplinary review. The Mental Health (Amendment) Act, which came into effect in 1982 moved some considerable way towards this position. Gostin and Mind thought it hadn't moved nearly far enough; some psychiatrists thought it had moved far too fast in the wrong direction. It was thus a classic British compromise. For the first time, it laid down in law that the consent of the patient to treatment was generally not required. This was decried by Gostin as a retrograde step that eroded the rights of the vulnerable mental patient. But, on the other hand, it stated that consent would have to be obtained for any surgical treatment, administration of medicine or electro-convulsive therapy. Some psychiatrists thought this was wrong. Both sides were horrified, although for quite different reasons, by complicated provisions and exceptions under this general principle. If a psychiatrist wants to do without the patient's consent to these procedures, he must obtain a second medical opinion from an independent doctor. There are, however, a number of exceptions to this rule. With certain specified procedures, however, such as psychosurgery, the consent of the patient is not enough. A second medical opinion has to be sought which will validate the competency of the consent and confirm that the proposed treatment should go ahead. Psychiatrists have complained bitterly that these provisions will make their practice of medicine far more difficult and that patients will suffer as a result. Gostin has complained that a second medical opinion, with all its qualifications, does not provide a sufficient safeguard for the patients' rights.

Nevertheless, for the first time in British law the principle has been laid down that at least for certain procedures, of an experimental, hazardous or irreversible nature, the consent of the mental patient can and should be sought, which is surely an enlightened step recognising the importance of autonomy of the individual.

Prisoners

Unlike the situation in the United States, there is unanimous agreement in this country that prisoners should not be used for non-therapeutic experiments on the grounds that there must always be a strong element of coercion or inducement within a prison. The problem arises over therapeutic experiments, because the same argument, that a prisoner's informed consent is invalid as a result of the pressures of prison life, applies. The problem has arisen mainly over prisoners requiring psychiatric treatment—sex offenders, for example, for whom psychosurgery might be considered appropriate. While such procedures were carried out on a few prisoners a few years ago, they have now been stopped on the grounds that a prisoner cannot, by definition, provide informed consent. It can be argued that a prisoner is in an analogous position to a mental patient detained under the Mental Health Act in that the mental patient is subject to similar coercive pressures in a similarly enclosed, restrictive environment. He too, it could be said, is prey to similar pressure to do the authorities' bidding.

Whatever the similarities, there does seem to be an important difference. The psychiatric hospital may be custodial, even punitive in practice but it is essentially a therapeutic institution. It undoubtedly serves the purpose of keeping mentally ill people away from society for its protection, and to that extent it is similar to a prison; but it has an overriding function which is to treat the mental

sickness of those within its walls. Thus, while there is a need
for stringent safeguards to ensure that consent to irreversible
procedures is valid, or that the overriding of consent is valid,
the underlying therapeutic nature of the institution makes
such procedures permissible.

A prison, however, is in no way a therapeutic institution,
even though it may contain an increasing number of mentally
sick inmates. Its medical facilities are undoubtedly stretched
to the limit in treating highly disturbed prisoners, or those
with chronic or terminal disease. But the structure of the
institution is not geared to the prisoner's best interests, in the
way that a hospital is. The underlying pressures upon a
prisoner must always undermine the validity of his consent.
The problem with this distinction between prison and
hospital, however, is as always the special hospitals. These,
as we have commented elsewhere, comprise a fatal confusion
between imprisonment and therapy, because they are in
essence prisons for the mad, subject to the same kind of
central government control and isolation from public scrutiny as the prison service.

Foetal research

The development of *in vitro* fertilisation (IVF) is one of the
clearest examples of medical science running far ahead of
morality, of scientific advances designed to benefit mankind,
and having enormous beneficial effects, bringing in their
train consequences so awesome and potentially terrible as to
prompt the question of whether the research should be
allowed to continue. The benefits of the technique are by
now obvious. Some 10 per cent of married couples suffer
from infertility, and many disorders causing such infertility
can now be bypassed by IVF, which involves fertilising an
egg outside the womb and then implanting the embryo in the
uterus. So far as the fundamental principle of the technique is
concerned, few people would cavil at the ethics of it. The
problems arise from secondary considerations. Is it acceptable to fertilise an egg with a donor sperm and then replace
the embryo in the womb, or fertilise a donor egg with the

husband's sperm? Is it acceptable to store or freeze embryos for future use? If so, is it acceptable for such embryos to be implanted in a mother who has no genetic relationship at all with the embryo? Is it acceptable for surrogate mothers to be used, in cases where a woman might be able to produce eggs but cannot undergo a pregnancy? Is it acceptable for 'spare' embryos to be killed or used as tissue for research?

This last problem is probably the most difficult to resolve, so let us look first at the other dilemmas arising from IVF (not that these are simple either). The repugnance caused by such possibilities in itself tends to be so great that one reaction is to cry halt to the whole programme on the grounds that we have swum into waters too deep for moral safety. This repugnance is caused by our deeply held feeling that man's new-found ability to create human life is essentially monstrous, despite the undoubted joy and benefit it brings to otherwise childless couples; that the manipulation of creation opens up possibilities of genetic programming that not so long ago belonged in the more nightmarish reaches of science fiction. But it is possible to think through the various dilemmas thrown up by IVF and isolate those consequences which seem acceptable and those which do not.

Two committees have now produced their own reports on these issues. The first, entitled 'Human Procreation: Ethical Aspects of the New Techniques' was produced by a working party of the Council for Science and Society. The second, more significant report was produced by the government-appointed committee of inquiry into human fertilisation and embryology which was chaired by the philosopher Dame Mary Warnock. Both reports steered clear, in the main, of the philosophical rocks that threatened their enterprise. The Council for Science and Society's report adopted a pragmatic approach, stating that its purpose was 'to facilitate thoughtful consideration and informed public discussion'. The Warnock report revealed that committee members were well aware of the deep divisions among different sections of society about the issues under consideration; indeed, the committee was unable to reach a unanimous view on two of the thorniest subjects, surrogate motherhood and research on embryos, and had to publish as a result two minority reports on these

particular matters. But the committee also recognised people's need and desire to set moral boundaries. 'People
generally want *some principles or other* to govern the development and use of the new techniques. There must be *some*
barriers that are not to be crossed, *some* limits fixed, beyond
which people must not be allowed to go. Nor is such a wish
for containment a mere whim of fancy. The very existence of
morality depends on it.'

Fertilisation with donor gametes
This is the easiest problem to solve, since in essence the
principles involved do not differ from those involved in
artificial insemination by donor, which has been accepted for
several years. Provided the embryo develops inside the
woman whose egg has been fertilised, or whose husband (or
partner) has provided the sperm, there would seem to be no
ethical objection.

Storage of embryos
The advantages of storing embryos are various. It would
enable the embryo to be replaced in the uterus in a cycle
uncomplicated by the administration of hormones. If multiple eggs were extracted, it would enable embryos to be
implanted in successive cycles until success was achieved. It
would enable women to plan pregnancies far later in life than
would be advisable, in view of the risk of developmental
defect, if late pregnancy were to occur naturally. But set
against these advantages is the risk that freezing and thawing
an embryo might harm it. And there is no way of finding out
whether such harm would occur without experimenting,
which would carry the distinct risk of damage to some of the
embryos tested. Damage to the embryo at any stage in these
circumstances is unacceptable, as we shall explain in our
section on 'spare' embryos. But in addition, storage would
carry the risk of delayed damage, not detectable until birth or
later in life. Such a risk would be far too high a price to pay
for the benefits of storage.

Implantation in an unrelated woman and surrogate mothers
It might be argued that, if one decides that storage of

embryos is unacceptable, the problem of whether or not to implant an embryo into a genetically unrelated woman becomes irrelevant. While it is true that prohibiting storage would probably reduce the possibility of such a transfer, it is not unthinkable that embryos could be implanted in unrelated women as quickly as they are implanted in the natural mother. Would this in itself be wrong? Ian Kennedy has argued that such a situation would be akin to the problem of the surrogate mother, and since he is opposed to surrogate motherhood he would prohibit implantation in an unrelated woman.

But it is far from clear that embryo donation is the same as surrogate motherhood. The problem with surrogate motherhood is not the legal position of the child, since this would be akin to the unsatisfactory legal position of children conceived by AID and as susceptible to law reform. The difficulty is more profound. It relates to the emotional bond that grows up during pregnancy between the mother and unborn infant. The surrogate mother runs an unacceptable risk that she will, by the time of the birth, strongly identify with the unborn child she has nourished and brought to life and feel it belongs to and is part of her. It is surely an abuse of a woman's body, even self-abuse, to treat the reproductive facility as a kind of greenhouse in which to grow a human from seed. Pregnancy and birth is a process in which a natural feature is a developing bond with the unborn child. It seems that to use a surrogate is to degrade the woman and potentially to disadvantage the child. However, this is one issue which has been left somewhat up in the air after the CSS and Warnock reports. For although both committees were in no doubt that surrogate motherhood was unsatisfactory and objectionable, there were disagreements over what to do about it. The CSS report concluded that however undesirable surrogate motherhood was, it should not be made illegal since it could be practised clandestinely and it could even be justified in very exceptional circumstances. This was broadly the conclusion reached by the dissenting minority on the Warnock committee, where the majority view held that although surrogacy itself should not be made illegal, since this would create criminals out of the mothers, it should be illegal for any agencies to bring about surrogacy arrangements. Our own view on this matter is that the majority on Warnock was right, and that the criminal law has to be used to prevent the risk of any commercial exploitation of surrogacy.

'Spare' embryos

The most important and difficult problem of all, however, is the dilemma of 'spare' embryos. It is here that we reluctantly part company with the majority on the Warnock committee. We have discussed in the chapter on life the controversy over where life begins, and have expressed our view that, although life is a continuum, fertilisation is the most significant marker along that process because it is from that point that human tissue becomes capable of growing and developing by itself into a person. Dr Robert Edwards, one of the team that pioneered IVF, disagrees with this analysis, arguing that the creation of life is a continuum and that no one stage counts as the beginning of life. He also contends that the embryo, at least for the first few days of its development, is a microscopic speck of tissue. Yet even he concedes that there are ethical problems associated with these specks:

Research on embryos raises questions about the fundamental rights of the human embryo—such questions as when life begins and whether embryos have any rights at all. The embryos I am discussing are minute: thousands could be included in a single drop. They are minute bundles of cells; they do not have hands or heads. They change into various unique shapes, none resembling a human being until seven weeks of gestation. Yet an obvious ethical situation arises concerning these minute specks of life, where the opportunities for good must be balanced against values of life.

This appears to be a muddled approach. On the one hand, Edwards is stressing the extreme smallness of the embryo as if to emphasise that they should not be treated like living beings; but on the other he is saying that all life forms pose ethical dilemmas.

It may be argued that as we permit abortions, there can be

no reason why we should prohibit research into, and the killing of, IVF embryos.

But as we have argued in our section on abortion, the taking of life in those circumstances is balanced against the various disadvantages of letting the pregnancy continue. Life, as we have seen, is not sacrosanct in our society but there do have to be overwhelming reasons for destroying it.

To create life, that potential for personhood, with the sole purpose of using it as experimental tissue before it is destroyed, undermines our respect for the uniqueness of human life. It can be argued that abortion has already undermined that respect, and to some extent we believe that to be true. But it is a matter of balance. We sanction abortions because we believe that the continuation of the pregnancy may be unacceptable for the mother. The consequence of prohibiting research on and the destruction of spare embryos would not cause such harm; it would only cause, at worst, the absence of a benefit.

Dr Edwards has raised two important points on this issue—one rather disingenuous, and the other much more powerful. His less useful point is that 'spare' embryos are the inevitable result of hormonal stimulation of the ovaries, necessary because implanting these embryos in the uterus significantly increases the chance of a successful pregnancy. But this is to elide two distinct parts of the IVF process. The production of extra eggs may indeed be inevitable through hormonal stimulation, but the existence of spare embryos is not inevitable at all; they can only be created if Dr Edwards deliberately fertilises them. It is possible, surely, for three eggs only to be fertilised. But that is where Dr Edwards's second point comes in. He has argued that experimenting on the 'spare' foetal tissue may provide valuable information about serious disorders and genetic mutations. In addition, such experimentation is presumably important in providing the most favourable conditions for those embryos that will eventually be implanted. Presumably, also, the greater the number of eggs fertilised *in vitro*, the greater the chance of a successful conception.

So in effect what we have to decide is this: is the destruction of this primitive life form justified if by doing so we reap a potential benefit to future generations of children, or promote the success of this particular fertilisation technique? We should be in no doubt what it is that is being destroyed—an embryo with a claim to life and all the potential of a genetically unique individual.

The Warnock committee was divided on this issue, but the majority concluded that research should be permitted on embryos of up to 14 days' gestation. They decided that the embryo should be afforded some protection in law because 'the embryo of the human species ought to have a special status'. But they decided that such protection should start at 14 days because that was just before the primitive streak started to appear which marked the beginning of individual development of the embryo. This, however, seems to be an arbitrary dividing line. As we have argued earlier, there are many milestones in the development of the human embryo, whose status changes during gestation. But it is hard to see why 'individual development' is any more significant than the moment when a single cell is created with a complete set of chromosomes which, all things being equal (which admittedly they often are not), will grow into a unique human being. It is impossible to reconcile a respect for human life if one is creating it with a view to using it as experimental material and then disposing of it. From the arguments of the majority on the Warnock committee, it appears more that members were aware of the need to respect life but equally did not want to lose the opportunities for research that would disappear under an outright ban. So they tried to reach the classic compromise. 'We do not want to see a situation', they wrote,

in which human embryos are frivolously or unnecessarily used in research but we are bound to take account of the fact that the advances in the treatment of infertility, which we have discussed in the earlier part of this report, could not have taken place without such research; and that continued research is essential, if advances in treatment and medical knowledge are to continue.

The dividing line, therefore, seems to have been drawn here with an eye to pragmatic expediency. While pragmatism and compromise are not to be sneered at, we feel that there are some values which, however awkward the consequences may be, are simply too important to take second place unless it is otherwise impossible to prevent harm. We feel that respect for human life is one of those values and that infertility, although a blight, is more an absence of good than an actual harm.

Genetic screening

We have already touched on some of the fundamental problems involved in genetic screening in our chapter on life. Part of the dilemma posed by this relatively recent advance in medical science relates to the question of when life begins and the sanctity or otherwise of the life of the foetus, discussed in the chapter on life, and above. But even if these problems are resolved to general satisfaction, other agonising dilemmas remain. Genetic abnormalities are often grave and lethal conditions which cannot be cured. Detecting them, or detecting the carriers of them, may generate terrible fear among relatives; the uncertainty of diagnosis may mean the loss of healthy children through abortion; a host of silent carriers may, through being identified, become prey to a variety of psychiatric disorders as a result. As its best, genetic counselling should simply provide people with the information to equip them to make decisions for themselves. The counsellor should not try to guide people towards a specific course of action, however much they might want the counsellor to do just that. Nevertheless, those decisions imposed on people by their new knowledge gained and disseminated in order to mitigate and minimise human suffering, may cause them supreme mental anguish. Moreover, it may be difficult for the counsellor to judge what to do to cause the least harm.

One of the most useful papers on the dilemmas of genetic screening was written in 1976 by A. Arnold and R. Moseley of the Department of Human Genetics and Biometry, University College, London. It is worth going into their arguments in some detail. They point out the difficulties for

the genetic counsellor in making an accurate diagnosis and
prediction of the recurrence of the disorder. For example, a
haemophiliac-carrying woman may not know whether she will
produce a haemophiliac child or not. When telling the
parents what the probability is, the counsellor may unconsciously weight his information by saying, variously, that
there is for example a 10 per cent chance of a defective child
or a 90 per cent chance of a normal child. Accordingly, argue
the authors, the counsellor should make both statements to
avoid bias. Then there is the problem of high risk relatives. If
it is clear that other relatives may be affected by the disorder
carried by the patient, should these relatives be told? The
authors draw a distinction between treatable, avoidable and
untreatable conditions. In the case of treatable or avoidable
diseases, they say, the counsellor should trace relatives at risk
and treat or advise them. But in cases of untreatable disease,
they say, relatives should not be told because this would
simply spread tremendous anxiety.

There is also the balance to be struck between the interests
of the individual and the interests of the community. Which
should be given preference? The birth of defective children
has consequences for the parents, for the child, for society
and for the human race. The authors comment:

The effect of a cure (for example, pyloric stenosis has been operated
on successfully over the past 50 years) or rise in living standards is
typically to change a condition that has formerly reduced survival
and so reduce natural selection against causative genes. The increase
in the frequency of the gene in the next generation is proportional
to the improvement in fitness brought about by treatment. . . .
Society may in some fashion have to place restrictions on
reproduction or make appropriate plans to allocate more resources
to disease in future generations, so we must decide how to manage
both to live humanely with genetic disease and at the same time to
conquer it.

Another problem relates to the likelihood of false positive
or false negative results. False negative results can mean that a
defective child slips through the screening net. False positive
results can mean that a healthy infant is mistakenly aborted.
In addition, there is the small but nevertheless significant risk

posed by amniocentesis itself, the removal for testing of amniotic fluid cells from the mother's uterus. Parents tend to consider more than this risk when deciding whether or not to have an amniocentesis; they consider the risk of serious and long-term handicap, whether the child would die early, whether the condition would be mild or whether treatment was available.

Such screening is primarily for the purpose of avoiding the birth of a handicapped baby. But, as the authors comment, a grave problem arises when genetic disease is identified in a living patient when there is no treatment available:

If the condition is chronic and progressive, as is muscular dystrophy of the Duchenne type, and no treatment is available, knowing about the condition before its manifestations may merely provoke anxiety both for the patient and for the parents. It could be argued that diagnosis of the genetic defect before the existence of overt disease infringes upon the ethical values of security for both parents and child. For, although prior knowledge of a defect supports the ethical value of telling the truth, it does so at the expense of other very important ethical values.

A particular example of these awful dilemmas is provided by the detection of Huntington's Chorea, which has been called the most serious genetic disorder of adult life in Western populations. The progressive physical and mental deterioration of the disease, coupled with the hereditary implications for relatives, places an often intolerable burden upon families. Each child of an affected person has a 50 per cent chance of inheriting the responsible gene but carriers can't be identified until there are clinical signs of the disease itself. By the time these appear, the carrier may have had children. So it is obviously important that the potential carrier is warned before having children. But what should such people be told? Segal has written:

Considering the possible mental anguish and the exceptionally high incidence of suicide in Huntington's families, the dilemma is whether it is humane and ethical to direct a young person's thoughts to the, at best (or worst) 50–50 chance that he or she might deteriorate into the condition witnessed in a relative, and should govern life accordingly. Thus, an individual who might never have consciously or otherwise contemplated the possibility of personal involvement might have life and hope blighted, and survival without development of the disease might be little compensation for a lifetime of anxiety, dread and single status.

Recently, the situation has developed further. There are signs that a predictive test may soon be available. This would carry the obvious advantage to society that carriers could be warned in advance not to have children, but it also carries the disadvantage of psychological damage to the carrier who is informed of his condition, and in the case of a young carrier with apparently normal parents, poses the additional dilemma of telling them whether they too are about to develop the disease. In other words, it is a classic example of the conflict between serving the interests of society and those of the individual. It is also an example of how one of the cardinal principles of medicine, telling the truth, can conflict with another principle, to do no harm.

Current limitations of technique themselves create dilemmas. For example, it is impossible to distinguish normal male foetuses from those suffering from sex-linked disease, as in haemophilia. So if all male foetuses at risk were aborted, at least half of them would have been normal. Similarly, raised alphafetoprotein level does not give a clear indication of the degree of neural tube defect that it detects, so routine abortion of such foetuses will involve the destruction of potentially salvageable children. As time goes on, however, it is reasonable to suppose that these screening techniques will become more and more sophisticated, thus diminishing the problems of inaccuracy. But, as Mason and McCall Smith comment:

increasing sophistication to some extent only serves to increase the fundamental moral issue of prenatal screening which is—how far is one to go in defining abnormality? The concept of parents obtaining a termination for frivolous reasons such as the sex of a child is obviously unacceptable, but one can foresee more plausible dilemmas of conscience. Cases of Down's Syndrome or of spina bifida which have not been discovered through prenatal screening are already candidates for neonaticide or local authority care. Is such disposal to run parallel with an increasing prenatal diagnostic capability when, as a result, more parents reject what will be regarded as imperfect children on increasingly demanding criteria?

Directing research

Underlying the whole discussion of the ethical dilemmas arising from research and experimentation lies the question: should we direct medical research? The question is likely to be received in some sections of the medical profession with considerable hostility, because it is a maxim among scientists as a whole that research should not be curbed in any way. But although the aims of many research projects are undoubtedly laudable, they tend to bring in their wake a host of hideous and often insoluble dilemmas.

Research tends not to bring unmitigated advantages, but to bring benefits which have to be set against disadvantages that it has created and which did not previously exist. In other words, research brings harm as well as good. Sometimes the harm may outweigh the good. One thinks of the disproportionate cost of heart transplantation, for example, which can distort the health budget to the detriment of many more people than the procedure helps. Or one thinks of the IVF programme, with its clouded moral waters. Is there not a case for trying to co-ordinate such research in the interests of a coherent view of society's goals? Is there not a case for a philosophy of medicine?

4
THE STATE

Behind many of the dilemmas of modern medicine lies a particular shadow—the memory of the Nazi period and in particular the role played by German doctors in the barbarities of that time. If the world stood aghast when the full horror of the Final Solution was eventually revealed, it was perhaps particularly sickened by the role of the doctors in the extermination programme and the perversion of medicine that this involved. The doctors were used in various ways. They conducted the medical experiments carried out on the prisoners of war and on those in the concentration camps. These experiments included testing existence at high altitudes by placing victims in a pressurised chamber and then lowering the pressure within it; freezing experiments, in which victims were kept in tanks of iced water or kept naked outdoors in freezing temperatures; infecting concentration camp inmates with malaria, hepatitis virus, or spotted fever; sulfanilamide experiments, in which wounds deliberately inflicted upon victims were then infected with bacteria or aggravated by having wood shavings or ground glass forced in them; poison experiments, in which victims were administered poison to see its effects. Doctors were also involved in euthanasia and sterilisation programmes and in the extermination procedures themselves. Many of these experiments resulted in death or grave injury to the victims. The medical knowledge gained was virtually worthless because, quite apart from the bestiality of these activities, they were conducted in secret and could not be reported or scrutinised. Without publication and discussion, the rigour of an experiment cannot be tested, the work cannot be repeated and the protocol remains unknown.

These horrors raised several crucial issues for the medical

profession. It had to face the fact that Nazi totalitarianism had been greatly facilitated by the application of science and technology and helped by the participation of the doctors. It had to face up to the evidence that the ethical traditions of medicine had not prevented German doctors from perverting their calling in these hideous ways, either by participating in these activities because they were themselves Nazis and believed in the Nazi objectives, or by allowing themselves to be coerced into participating and by failing to resist. Either way, their culpability was evident. In the decades that followed the Nuremberg Trials in which these crimes were documented, the shadow of these awful events has fallen over a great many scientific developments and movements in social policy. The arguments over abortion or euthanasia, for example, or the treatment of the mentally handicapped, or the selective treatment of handicapped babies, or genetic counselling—all are conducted against the fearful insistence that we must never slide down the slippery slope to another Final Solution. And behind all these individual issues and the parallels that are drawn with Nazi ideology lies another, even greater issue—the relationship between doctors and the state. Those German doctors who were not themselves Nazi supporters but who nevertheless took part in, or failed to stop the scientific application of Nazism allowed themselves, sometimes by a quite gradual and subtle process, to be sucked into this perversion of their profession. If they had united in protest, refusal, resistance, they might have stopped much of what happened. So, fifty years on from the Third Reich, should doctors pay the closest attention to laws which might require them to infringe their ethical duties? Should they protest and organise against such developments, and if they fail to prevent them from taking place, what should they do? In a democracy, are they justified in breaking the law? Do medical ethics require doctors, on occasion, to consider themselves above the law? How far should they participate in activities required by the state which they think are wrong, in order to minimise inevitable suffering? And in deciding such issues, how useful is the Nazi experience as a warning analogy anyway?

Although the German experience undoubtedly affected

post-war thinking in medical ethics, there are those who question the extent to which it is relevant. The issue was discussed in 1976 at a conference in the United States on the proper use of the Nazi analogy in ethical debate. Much modern fearfulness about issues such as euthanasia, sterilisation, and medical experiments derives from our revulsion at the way in which these processes were used in Nazi Germany. But just because, during that time, sterilisation and euthanasia were performed to generate the pure *Volk*, the master race, and medical experiments were a form of torture, it does not necessarily follow that similar abuses will inevitably follow from the same processes in a modern democracy. The American conference pointed out correctly that the Nazi regime was uniquely wicked. There is a danger in drawing too close a parallel with that era. Nevertheless, certain lessons can be learnt from that time.

For example, Professor Joel Colton, a historian, argued that in all totalitarian dictatorships, the freedom of silence did not exist.

I think that one of the most serious things that one can say about the scientific community, and by extension the research community and academic community in Germany, is not that it didn't throw itself into some kind of political effort to stop Nazism, but that it did not even protest when the government itself began to interfere with universities and tell them what to do. The scientists accepted this; and then step by step some of them went down the path to very active cooperation.

How many doctors were enthusiastic co-operators remains a matter of some doubt. But it is more useful for the modern, democratic doctor to look at the position of those doctors who were not enthusiastic supporters of the regime but went along with its excesses nevertheless. The conference heard about a book by a pseudonymous German called Peter Bamm, entitled *The Invisible Flag*. It was about a German surgeon who had 'fled' into the German 11th Army, in an attempt to avoid the difficult situation back home, only to find that he was helping round up Jews for extermination. He wrote:

A few months later the 11th Army captured Sevastopol, whereupon all the Jewish inhabitants were collected and put to death in special poison vans. We knew all this, yet we did nothing. If anyone had protested or undertaken some positive action against the murder squad, he would have been arrested twenty-four hours later and would have disappeared. It is one of the most ingenious stratagems of the totalitarian system that they gave their opponents no opportunity to die a martyr's death for their convictions. For this there would have been no shortage of candidates. But a man who chose this death, rather than the silent toleration of such atrocities, would have sacrificed his life in vain. I do not of course imply that such self-sacrifice would have been useless in a moral sense. I am only saying that as a practical measure it would have been pointless.

This may well have been the case at that late stage and in those specific circumstances. But it might have been quite different had the challenge been made to the state at the beginning of the tyranny. If every single doctor had resisted and refused to participate in mass murder, then possibly this would have had some effect. As Professor Telford Taylor, chief counsel for the prosecution at the Nuremberg Trials, said:

the medical profession, like the legal profession, like engineering and many others, is highly organised; and these organisations were the vehicles through which Nazi demands were made and which rendered unavoidable a collective response. Almost uniformly, of course, the response was to succumb and to go along.

But if the collective response was unavoidable, the doctors did not have to succumb. Their collective response could have been resistance. And indeed, as Professor Dawidowicz pointed out, there were some doctors who did exactly that:

We know that there were German physicians who refused to participate in the 'euthanasia' programme and asked to be excused. And there's some evidence that they resigned or withdrew from that particular programme without suffering reprisals. So there was, at least in some areas, the possibility to refuse. It may be that in many places a lot of pressure was exerted to keep the medical professionals in line. And of course people had to make choices between career and non-career, comfort and non-comfort. Some Germans, we know, exercised such options.

When it came to consideration of the individual 'scientific' activities of the Nazis and their lessons for medical ethics, opinions were divided. The conference was told that the so-called 'euthanasia' programme was launched after the father of a deformed infant asked Hitler's permission to have his child killed. Thus, opponents of euthanasia have argued that since the Nazi attitude towards the incurable sick was the 'infinitely small, wedged-in level' that provided the impetus for mass murder, mercy killing should not be legalised. But Professor Dawidowicz argued that the analogy was irrelevant because the Nazi attitude towards euthanasia was never grounded in concern for medical problems but was always geared to the racialist Nazi ideology of the *Volk*. This in itself does not seem an irrefutable argument. As Milton Himmelfarb of the American Jewish Committee pointed out, the notion of social utility did figure in Nazi ideology as part of the *Volkisch* racism. 'You can still say it is fairly likely that a dictator, not necessarily a racist but obsessed by his notions of social utility, will use a term such as "non-rehabilitable" to mean, "Get rid of 'em, because the the cost exceeds the benefit." ' Or as another conference participant argued, the redefinition of political opponents as 'sick' rang a bell with those who were concerned about the use and abuse of medical categories to identify and label social deviants.

In other words, for an analogy to be appropriate it is not necessary for situations to be identical in every respect. As Laurence McCullough, a post-doctoral fellow at the Hastings Centre for ethical research, said:

Our slippery slope might yet be analogous to Nazi Germany's in a more abstract way. If we consider the rationale which gives social utility or economic returns precedence over individual freedom, then we might see how our society could approach the kind of thinking that underlay the Nazi experience. There, racism overrode personal autonomy; here, it might be an economic rationale—the attitude that we won't spend so much per year to keep somebody alive on the slim chance of recovery. The slippery slope, then, is not the precipitating act; it's the context in which that act takes place.

From that point of view, it would seem appropriate to have the Nazi experience in mind when considering the relationship between the doctor and the state, as a warning against the way in which doctors may be sucked into a state policy which absolutely negates their ethical codes. The Nazi experience showed how the collective response of the medical profession provided the mechanics of repression, how it was possible for doctors to resist the system without reprisals, how the doctors taking part in the repression (who weren't themselves Nazis) chose passive coercion instead. Unique as the Nazi terror was, those lessons for doctors are instructive today in a world where, unfortunately, murder, torture and ill-treatment by the state are a commonplace.

Torture

What is torture?

The dictionary definition is simple. Torture is the deliberate infliction of pain in order to extract a confession or to act as a punishment. But as Leonard Sagan and Albert Jonsen have pointed out, various thinkers have concluded that torture has a wider meaning.

The Amnesty International Committee convened to study the matter points out that torture has a number of essential facets that expand the definition. At least two persons must be involved, the torturer and his victim. Secondly, the victim is under the physical control of the torturer. Thirdly, although infliction of pain is a basic element, the definition must also include the essential feature of mental or psychological stress. Fourthly, there is an implicit intent on the part of the torturer to break the will of the victim, to destroy his humanity. Jean-Paul Sartre has written that the purpose of torture is 'not only the extortion of confessions of betrayal, but the victim must disgrace himself by his screams and his submission like a human animal. In the eyes of everybody and in his own eyes, he who yields under torture is not only to be made to talk but is also to be marked as sub-human.' Solzhenitsyn also writes, 'Of all forms of oppression, it is the practice of torture which most

relentlessly seeks to disintegrate the fundamental freedom of
human personality. Firstly, by naked assault and degradation and
secondly by attempts to gain absolute control over the victim's
will.

When international protocols and conventions talk about
torture, they use the word to convey a rather wider meaning
than the techniques of beating, burning, racking, electric
shocks or other physical mutilation generally associated with
the term. Torture is used to cover inhuman or degrading
treatment as well. Article Six of the Declaration of Torture of
the UN, 1975, reads: 'Torture constitutes an aggravated or
deliberate form of cruel, inhuman or degrading treatment or
punishment.' Some capital may be made out of the distinction between torture and other forms of ill-treatment. When
the European Court of Human Rights found the United
Kingdom guilty of ill-treatment in Northern Ireland but not
guilty of torture, *The Times* berated the Dublin government
for having tried to prove that Britain had tortured people.
Such an attitude is a little hard to understand, especially since
the British government admitted in its submissions that its
behaviour had amounted to torture or inhuman treatment,
according to the UN definition. In any event, and especially
in the context of medical ethics, the distinction makes no
difference to the morality of such behaviour. Inhuman or
degrading treatment, while not necessarily amounting to
torture, is indefensible.

The scale of the problem

Ever since the proclamation in 1948 of the Universal
Declaration of Human Rights, international instruments
condemning torture have multiplied. Yet, so far from
receding, torture has, in the words of Amnesty International
and the International Committee of the Red Cross, spread
like a cancer across the world. Eric Martin, the former
President of the ICRC, has commented that torture is not the
remnant of a barbaric age destined to disappear with the
progress of civilisation.

Virtually eliminated from European states by the end of the 19th
century, it has come back in full force, even within nations that

claim to be in the forefront of social and legal progress . . . Modern techniques, derived from a misuse of science, increase the cruelty and horror of the methods of torture used. Under medical supervision, the processes used can be continued and intensified, their cruelty and virulence increased, without killing the victims. In some states torture actually constitutes a method of governing; in others, the use of torture is common and widely tolerated. A doctor knows the physical and psychological pain caused by illnesses or accidents, by cancer which spreads throughout the body, by certain illnesses of the nervous system; he is often able to relieve this suffering, and tries to do just that. A torturer creates pain instead of reducing it; he intensifies and maintains it.

The problem is that despite the various protocols and conventions outlawing torture, the practice persists; despite their ethical injunctions to the contrary, doctors continue to play a part in it. In 1980 Mr Alfred Gellhorn, the immediate past president of the Council for International Organisations of the Medical Sciences, wrote despairingly to *The Lancet*:

The conviction at the Nuremberg Trials of some of those doctors and nurses who carried out atrocious 'experiments' on concentration camp inmates during the third Reich was based on their actions which were 'contrary to usages established among civilised people, to the laws of humanity and to the dictates of public conscience'. One outcome of the trials was the Nuremberg code—ten principles which, with elaborations, have guided human experimentation throughout the world. Nowadays, many countries have totalitarian regimes, and repression of human and civil rights is commonplace. Along with the suppression of dissension, torture has frequently become state policy, a spreading social cancer, as Amnesty International has characterised it. And once again evidence has accumulated which implicates the health professions in torture and other 'cruel, degrading and inhuman treatment of prisoners and detainees'.

In 1975, the World Medical Association adopted the Declaration of Tokyo which laid down guidelines for doctors relating to torture during detention or imprisonment. This said:

The doctor shall not countenance, condone or participate in the practice of torture or other forms of cruel, inhuman or degrading procedures whatever the offence of which the victim is suspected, accused or guilty, and whatever the victim's beliefs or motives, and in all situations including armed conflict or strife.

The declaration emphasised the doctor's role as a healer, and forbade doctors to facilitate torture or diminish the victim's ability to resist, or to be present while any such procedure was used or threatened, or to force-feed prisoners refusing food. But even this declaration was not watertight. For example, it did not prohibit doctors from examining victims before and after torture; indeed, by emphasising 'the doctor shall in all circumstances be bound to alleviate the distress of his fellow men', it could be interpreted to mean that a doctor is bound to play just such a role. In 1978, the WHO asked the Council for International Organisations of the Medical Sciences and the World Medical Association to draft a code for medical ethics relevant to torture, which supplemented the Declaration of Tokyo. This laid down that prisoners and detainees have the same rights to treatment as free citizens; that it was a contravention of medical ethics for a physician to have any other purpose than to improve or protect the health of the prisoner or detainee in the sense that this would be accepted outside the prison environment, and that therefore it would be wrong for doctors to certify prisoners or detainees as fit for any form of punishment that may adversely affect physical or mental health. In his letter to *The Lancet*, Alfred Gellhorn recognised that such codes of guidance would have little impact upon sadistic or fanatical health professionals who welcomed opportunities to participate in torture. 'But to the vast majority of health professionals, it is hoped that this will increase their awareness of the existing "social cancer" of torture and their ability to withstand any request to become party to the unethical practices involved.' Unfortunately, there is as yet little sign of a wholesale worldwide revolt by health professionals against these odious practices in which they are involved.

Is torture ever justified?
To many people, the question will seem outrageous. Torture

arouses such deep feelings of revulsion among most people that the idea of deliberately inflicting pain and humiliation on a fellow human being is unthinkable. That is because we associate torture with repressive regimes, where the aims behind such suffering are themselves vile and reprehensible, and where the infliction of pain is enjoyed by those who practise it. But it is possible to conceive of circumstances in which torture might be contemplated for benign, even elevated reasons. Suppose, for example, terrorists had stolen a nuclear weapon and were threatening to explode it in a British city. Suppose one of them had been captured, but since there was no time to find the weapon, the only hope of saving the city lay in torturing the terrorist. Wouldn't the cause of saving millions of lives greatly outweigh the revulsion at torturing the terrorist? In other words, wouldn't the end justify the means? If it could be proved beyond doubt that torture was the only way of preventing such a catastrophe, the argument might apply. But all existing evidence points to the opposite conclusion—that torturing a suspect who would, in these circumstances, probably be trained and determined and prepared to die anyway would be counter-productive. Moreover, if torture were permissible to stave off a nuclear calamity the line could not be drawn there. What about a situation in which a far smaller number of people were in danger of being killed by a small conventional bomb? If the principle has been conceded for a great disaster, is it likely that the state would, or could, shrug its shoulders at a lesser one?

We pay a price for what we call our civilisation. Part of the gain we achieve from belonging to a civilised society is a feeling of moral superiority to those who seek to achieve their ends using violence. If we use unrestrained violence and torture to maintain our society, how do we differ from those who seek to subvert it? What complaint could we make if the boot were on the other foot and the authors of terrorist attacks controlled the machinery of the state and were then responsible for the organisation of society? The deaths and injuries that we suffer by our restraint are the price that we pay for something that we hold to be valuable.

The role of the physician

I'm thrown to the ground in the cell. It's hot. My eyes are blindfolded. The door opens and someone says that I'm to be moved. Two days have gone by without torture. The doctor came to see me and removed the blindfold from my eyes. I asked him if he wasn't worried about my seeing his face. He acts surprised. 'I'm your friend. The one that takes care of you when they apply the machine. Have you had something to eat?'

'I have trouble eating. I'm drinking water. They gave me an apple.'

'You're doing the right thing. Eat lightly. After all, Gandhi survived on much less. If you need something, call me.'

'My gums hurt. They applied the machine to my mouth.'

He examines my gums and advises me not to worry, I'm in perfect health. He tells me he's proud of the way I withstood it all. Some people die on their torturers, without a decision having been made to kill them; this is regarded as a professional failure. He indicates that I was once a friend of his father's, also a police doctor. His features do seem familiar. I mention his father's name; this is indeed the son. He assures me that I'm not going to be killed. I tell him that I haven't been tortured for two days and he's pleased.

This extract is taken from Jacobo Timerman's account of his imprisonment and torture by the Argentinian junta in the late 1970s. It illustrates well one of the parts doctors play in such procedures, and further illuminates the ambivalent attitudes on the part of such a physician—it is not clear whether this doctor is an enthusiast for the regime or not. What is clear is that he is an integral part of the proceedings. He has not come in response to Timerman's distress, but to make sure that he is in good enough shape to survive the next bout of torture, to make sure that he will not die on them and become a 'professional failure'. His role, as he presents it, is that of the prisoner's 'friend'—but it is a role that is central to the theatre of repression.

To that extent, the presence of the doctor in these proceedings was wholly wrong. But in some cases the dividing line between what is the right or wrong course of action for the doctor to take is less obvious—indeed, as the *Medical Journal of Australia* put it, it can pose an intolerable dilemma for the physician.

Unless he is utterly bereft of the humane attitudes taken for granted in our profession, he will have little hesitation in refusing to participate actively in the infliction of anything in the way of torture, even though here borderline situations arise. But the position is more difficult when his role appears to be the protection of the subject—the giving of medical aid, if necessary, or the advising of when the interrogation or punishment is becoming too much to be borne. This may be seen as a necessary and humane role—if it is not seen as a safeguard for those doing the interrogation or inflicting the punishment, a means of indicating how far they can go without killing the subject or a device for reviving the subject so that the process can go on. For the conscientious and humane doctor, the decision about what to do or what not to do can be bewildering.

There would, therefore, appear to be a clear distinction to be drawn between the doctor acting on behalf of the prisoner and at his request, and acting on behalf of the administration. In the former role, the doctor is acting entirely properly in attending to need and alleviating distress; in the latter, however, he is not only part of the process that is causing the distress but by virtue of his professional standing he is lending that process some spurious respectability since he appears to condone it—and furthermore, is making the process more efficient by ensuring that the victim doesn't die before it is finished. The problem is that in practice it is extremely difficult to separate the two. Examining a prisoner before he is tortured is more straightforward, since the only reason for such an examination is to pronounce the prisoner fit to undergo duress and therefore must be wrong. But examining the prisoner afterwards provokes the dilemma, since it could be in the prisoner's interest or in the interest of the torturers—in theory, at least. In practice, however, it is extremely unlikely that any doctor allowed to examine a prisoner in such circumstances would be a free agent, and that his treatment and opinion would not be used by the torturers.

The British experience

There is ample evidence of collusion by doctors around the

world in torture, and evidence of doctors themselves being tortured when they refuse to toe the government line. For example, Dr Sheila Cassidy, a British physician in Chile, was arrested, blindfolded, strapped naked to a metal bunk and tortured with electric shocks because she had treated those who had fallen out of favour with the government. In the Soviet Union, doctors sign the death certificates of those who have died from torture so that they appear to have died from natural causes. In Chile again, drugs such as cyclophosphamide have been used as part of a torture programme. But although such terrible and systematic abuses do not happen in the Western democracies, it would be wrong to imagine that the kind of dilemmas arising from the abuse of state power and the ill-treatment of prisoners do not happen here. Indeed, just such a problem erupted in Northern Ireland in the 1970s.

It was revealed that detainees who had not been convicted of any crime were being starved, deprived of sleep, made to stand spreadeagled against a wall for hours at a time—in one case, for as much as forty-three and a half hours in six days—hooded and exposed to continuous noise for long periods of time. A committee of inquiry was set up, headed by Sir Edward Compton, whose report eventually claimed that such methods of interrogation being used in Northern Ireland were not brutal. They were used to stop internees from communicating with each other, said the report, and in some cases to increase their sense of isolation and so be helpful to the interrogator. This was, many thought, a remarkable judgement. One person who was deeply shocked by this interpretation was the psychiatrist, Dr Anthony Storr. In 1973, he explained how he had written an article for *The Sunday Times* on the psychiatric aspects of the Compton Report because he realised that the general public would be unaware that psychological pressure without actual physical torture could nevertheless produce serious effects upon the victim. Dr Storr wrote in his 1973 account:

The hooding and the continuous noise were designed not to isolate men from each other but as a deliberate method of producing mental disorientation and confusion. I was not an expert in this field, but I knew that the effects were so disturbing that even a high proportion of healthy volunteers who were acting as experimental guinea pigs and being paid pressed the panic button long before the experiment was up. In conditions of mild sensory deprivation, many volunteers endured only an average of 29 hours, and in more rigorous conditions only one man in ten endured more than ten hours. If no time limit is set to such experiments, fears of insanity and confusion may come on within as little as two hours.

Dr Storr repeated his warning to the Parker committee which had been set up to investigate the matter further. But nevertheless Lord Parker and Mr John Boyd-Carpenter produced a majority report which endorsed these interrogation methods, subject to certain safeguards. It was left to Lord Gardiner, the third member of the committee, to demolish the majority conclusions in a dissenting minority report which said that such ill-treatment of suspects was wholly wrong, morally unjustifiable and illegal. Fortunately, his conclusions were accepted by the British government and these interrogation methods were then forbidden. But if Lord Gardiner had not been on that committee, or if the British government had chosen instead to heed the majority report, doctors would have been placed in serious ethical difficulties.

If interrogation does impose a strain on a person—as we may suppose—the argument is readily advanced that the attention of a doctor before such an ordeal is more humane than his absence, for presumably if the doctor pronounces the person medically unfit for interrogation it would not be carried out. Yet a slippery slope lies before us. Without ever becoming a participant in the interrogation, a doctor could, if he were automatically required to examine every prisoner before the interrogation started, come to be regarded as a part of the process and as sanctioning it in medical terms. For a captive to call for the aid of a doctor is one thing; for his captors to require a report from the doctor is another.

Such anxieties were greatly heightened by one of the 'safeguards' proposed in the majority report. This was to be the constant presence in the interrogation centre of a doctor with some psychiatric training who:

should be in a position to observe the course of oral interrogation. It is not suggested that he should be himself responsible for stopping the interrogation—rather that he should warn the controller if he felt that the interrogation was being pressed too far. . . . This should be some safeguard for the constitutionally vulnerable detainee and at the same time for the interrogator.

But what was 'too far'? A broken limb? Unconsciousness? Chronic depression? The report did not say. Nor did it concern itself with the ethics of a doctor sanctioning degrees of ill-treatment. Others, however, were extremely alarmed, even though Lord Gardiner's strictures had been accepted by the government. *The Lancet*, for example, commented:

Regrettably, the use of these techniques cannot be regarded as an aberration which can be relegated to oblivion. The very fact that brutal treatment was meted out for so long in so many countries, with so many (including *The Lancet*) ignorant or heedless of what was going on, underlines the need for doctors to learn from the past and to establish a firm line for the future. Doctors . . . should have no truck with the methods described by Compton. Firstly, these are incompatible with the standards which hold the profession together, and secondly (if a more mundane reason is needed) medical attendance at intensive interrogation can only lend the proceedings a gloss of restraint and of scientific insight which they do not merit.

There is a delicate path relating to a person's detention and which is designed to protect the prisoner from ill-treatment. The path steers clear of connivance in this way. Everyone who is detained undergoes a medical examination at the end of which a doctor pronounces impartially upon the prisoner's state of health—not whether he is 'fit' for questioning, but simply whether or not he is healthy. The doctor will recommend treatment for any clinical disease that he may detect. This examination creates a baseline record of the prisoner's condition at the time at which he was taken into detention. The record would provide valuable help to the prisoner if he were then to be ill-treated; but there is no medical collusion with any ill-treatment that may be inflicted. This procedure was the substance of advice given to

the Ministry of Defence by Dr Michael Thomas, the former
chairman of the BMA's Central Ethical Committee, and
which is now in force.

   The conclusions that society drew from this whole episode
were that ill-treatment of suspects was an abomination, and
that it was not impressed by the argument that such
ill-treatment of a few suspects might save a great many
lives—the argument presented by the Parker committee to
Dr Storr when he gave evidence to it. Lord Gardiner did not
spell out the moral reasons why he could not countenance
such ill-treatment. He simply said firmly:

I do not believe that, whether in peace time for the purpose of
obtaining information relating to men like the Richardson gang or
the Kray gang, or in emergency terrorist conditions, or even in war
against a ruthless enemy, such procedures are morally justifiable
against those suspected of having information of importance to the
police or army, even in the light of any marginal gain which may
thereby be obtained.

   In other words, for Lord Gardiner, at least, no ends can
justify such uncivilised means. Torture or the brutal treatment of detained persons corrupts society and brings its
administration down to the level of the violence it is trying to
eradicate. Any claim to moral authority made by a society is
destroyed in these circumstances and observers can only
watch dispassionately to see who, possessing the greater
force, will win the struggle.

   Had Lord Gardiner's views not prevailed, doctors would
have found themselves in the uncomfortable position of
being accessories to ill-treatment sanctioned by the state; they
would then have been torn between their ethical principles
and their duties to a democratic society. In fact, some years
later they were caught in just such a dilemma, again in
Northern Ireland. In January 1977, the Royal Ulster Consta-
bulary re-took control of the security situation in Northern
Ireland. Almost immediately, allegations began to surface
concerning the ill-treatment of detainees by police at Cast-
lereagh interrogation centre, and the bulk of these allegations
emanated from police surgeons or, as they are known in
Northern Ireland, Forensic Medical Officers.

The police surgeon

The police surgeon is in an exceptionally delicate position. He is usually employed by the police on a part-time basis to act as an impartial and expert examiner. Although he is paid by the police for his work, he is not their agent; the police may ask him to submit a report to them, but his examination must be carried out with the consent of the suspect or prisoner. In other words, since this is not a normal therapeutic relationship but one in which the information gathered by the doctor is used for purposes other than the patient's clinical care, the patient may very properly want to limit the information he discloses in the examination. In addition, however, the police doctor may be asked to examine and treat ill suspects in custody, in which case he forms a normal therapeutic relationship with the prisoner/ patient. So the police surgeon not only has to cope with two distinct functions within his role—he has to preserve his independence from his employer, the police, whose aims are quite different from his.

The aims of the police are, after all, to prevent and detect crime and bring offenders to justice. These are not the doctor's aims, and he must be careful not to be compromised. For example, if the police wanted the doctor to physically examine a suspect for signs of drug addiction and the suspect refused, the doctor would be breaching his ethical duty if he carried out the examination nevertheless—indeed, he would be committing an assault. If the suspect were unconscious and the doctor examined him, it would likewise be improper for any specimens or tests to be used for forensic purposes without his consent. As one police surgeon, Dr Stanley Burges, wrote in 1980:

It is acknowledged by police and police surgeons alike that a partial police surgeon is a liability to society, an embarrassment to his profession, and an encumbrance to the employing police authority. An expression of this impartiality is seen in Northern Ireland where, in spite of his time-honoured title, the police surgeon is now known as a Forensic Medical Officer.

And it was in Northern Ireland that this impartiality was put to its most severe and spectacular test. In 1979, the Bennett report revealed that the allegations of brutality were true and that most of the evidence had come from the police surgeons. One of these police surgeons, Dr Robert Irwin, appeared on television shortly before the report was published to say that he personally had examined between 150 and 160 people who had been ill-treated by about 20 detectives. Dr Irwin's allegations caused a furore, and he became the target of a whispering campaign about his qualifications and the state of his mental health. There were suspicions that the smears had originated in the Northern Ireland Office, although this was vehemently denied. But when the Bennett report was published, Dr Irwin was vindicated, and it became clear that he and his colleagues had played a substantial part in bringing these practices to light. The report said:

The forensic medical officers, early in 1977, examining prisoners at the stage when they were being charged at police stations throughout the province, noted in some police stations and police offices a large increase of significant bruising, contusions and abrasions of the body and evidence of hyper-extension and hyper-flexion of joints (especially of the wrists), of tenderness associated with hair pulling and persistent jabbing, of rupture of the ear drums and increased mental agitation and anxiety states. These officers, in the light of their own experience, were well aware of the need for caution in dealing with prisoners' complaints, and of the possibilities of exaggeration, invention and self-inflicted injury.

This would appear to be an example of doctors scrupulously observing their ethical principles, of acting independently and refusing to become parties to ill-treatment. Faced with the situation they perceived, they had only one way of stopping the ill-treatment and that was by making such activities publicly known. This would appear to vindicate a comment made by Dr Burges on a recommendation in the British Medical Association's *Handbook of Medical Ethics*. This says:

It is unethical for a doctor to carry out an examination on a person before that person is interrogated under duress or torture. Even though the doctor takes no part in the interrogation or torture, his examination of the patient prior to interrogation could be interpreted as condoning it.

But Dr Burges comments:

Events in Northern Ireland do not entirely support this view. Forensic Medical Officers there initiated the concept of the pre-interrogation medical examination on the grounds that an examination by an impartial and competent doctor before and after interrogation would make it possible to ascertain the truth of what happened in the intervening period. Thus, far from condoning torture, it would be an active means of exposing and preventing it. If, on the other hand, the intent is to assess fitness for torture, then, of course, it would be quite unacceptable, but this can easily be avoided if the results of the examination remain privy to the examiner.

This, however, is a big 'if'. If this were to happen as Dr Burges outlines, with the results of the examination privy to the doctor, then quite clearly the doctor would retain his independence and would in no way be colluding with unethical practices—quite the reverse. But given that he is actually employed by the police, who were committing the ill-treatment, it is hard to see how he could comfortably refuse to make the information known to them. If the police pressurised him to do what they wanted, and if he was unable to expose what was happening and thus prevent it, he would have no alternative but to resign. Something like this appears to have happened to Dr Denis Elliott, who for two years was the senior medical officer at Gough barracks, the interrogation centre in Armagh. Dr Elliott's position was even more difficult than that of Dr Irwin and the police surgeons, since he was a civil servant on secondment to the police authority. Thus he was a full-time employee of the state, and he was bound by the Official Secrets Act. Dr Irwin requested that Dr Elliott should be released from his duty of silence under the Act, but since this did not happen we don't know exactly what troubled Dr Elliott so much. What is a matter of public record, however, is that Dr Elliott resigned from his post at

Armagh barracks because he could not resolve the contradictions of his position. He said:

I have withdrawn because I have found it impossible to comply with the requirements of the Tokyo Convention of 1975 which deals with the conduct of medical officers in relation to prisoners under their care. I have taken satisfaction in the fact that there have not been any significant complaints at Gough barracks in eleven months.

Dr Elliott lacked the safety valve of disclosure that is available to police surgeons and which enables them to tread the delicate tightrope of their professional duties. However, there is always the risk that the state will add to those duties in a way that doctors find unacceptable. This happened with the Police and Criminal Evidence Act which remains a matter of acute controversy. Among its provisions, the Act permits an intimate search of a person in police custody who is suspected of having concealed a weapon or dangerous drug. The prisoner would have no opportunity to refuse such a search, but could ask for it to be performed by a doctor—and it would fall to the police surgeon to fulfil that duty. Some doctors protested at this provision, on the grounds that medical examinations should never be carried out without the consent of the patient, and that to carry out a forcible body search would constitute an assault and was thus totally unacceptable. However, the case was put even more forcibly by Dr Michael Wilks, a London GP and a police surgeon. In a letter to the *Guardian*, he criticised the British Medical Association for 'dangerous ambivalence' on the issue and for failing to understand the subtle but crucial way in which the provision would change the relationship between doctors and patients, doctors and the state.

There were three levels of objection to the provision. One was that forcible examination was unacceptable. The next objection was, however, that it was wrong to imply that consent to such an examination could make it acceptable, since true consent in such circumstances was unlikely. Apart from any element of coercion, a prisoner was likely, when faced with a choice between police officer and doctor, to choose the doctor—but that didn't mean that the consent was free and informed. The final objection was the most fundamental of all. Dr Wilks wrote:

the normal role of a doctor assisting the police, which is as an impartial expert, responsible to the police but conducting medical examinations with the consent of the subject, during the course of which evidence may be obtained and passed to the police. By writing doctors into a procedure in which a person is searched only for evidence, the doctor's role becomes one of an agent acting on behalf of the police. . . . This change in the responsibility of the medical profession marks the start of a long road at the end of which South African doctors are involved in interrogation and Russian doctors enter dissidents in psychiatric hospitals.

Dr Wilks was drawing a distinction between a doctor searching for evidence and examining a suspect's state of health. But since, in the context of a police surgeon's work, the health examination is done on behalf of the police, doesn't this count as an examination for a non-medical reason? Perhaps the answer is that there is a difference between a medical examination, i.e. one carried out to discover the state of a person's health, and then given by arrangement to the police, and a search which has got nothing to do with health at all. Indeed, one of the objections to the forcible body search is that you don't need a doctor to do it. True, a doctor would ensure that the suspect wasn't hurt or damaged by the procedure, which might happen if it were carried out by a police officer. And it might be argued that it is the doctor's duty to society to conduct such a search—for example, it has been suggested that a situation might arise in which a suspect was thought to have a detonator up his backside. (In practice, however, there would seem little point in a forcible search to get it out; all one would need to do would be to seclude the suspect in a room with a lavatory, and wait.) More commonly, a doctor might be asked to search for drugs hidden in the vagina. Even if free consent were given (which, as we have said, is extremely unlikely), if a doctor were to agree to do this he would be acting as no more than a retrieval service for the police. No clinical or diagnostic skills would be required at all.

A more sophisticated argument has been used to justify the involvement of doctors in forcible body searches. Supposing, it is said, a suspect is believed to have secreted a knife up his backside, with which he might either kill himself or another. Isn't it the doctor's duty, if requested by the police, to retrieve such a weapon in the cause of removing a threat to life? The answer, however difficult it might be to give in the police station, must surely still be no. The principle must be upheld that medical examinations should not be performed without free and informed consent. Forcible examination is not the same as removing someone's belt or shoelaces—it is an assault, and moreover a procedure for which there would appear to be no absolute necessity. The arguments against waiting and watching the suspect until the weapon emerges naturally are merely bureaucratic—not enough time or manpower, too much trouble, and so on. Moreover, if the doctor were to retrieve the knife, the weapon could be used as evidence against the suspect. So, under the ethical umbrella of preventing harm, the doctor would in fact be acting as an agent of the state in providing evidence for a criminal trial. Moreover, being told that someone might have a secret weapon which might be used against himself or someone else is hopelessly vague and uncertain. What if it is a domestic murderer who has in this way hidden the weapon with which he killed his wife? Just because the weapon is there does not necessarily mean he presents a danger to anyone else. What if a doctor fishes around for a knife but actually discovers a packet of heroin? If doctors were to accept that it was ethically proper to assault someone for the greater good of society, they could indeed be set on Dr Wilks's road to the Gulag.

As Dr Michael Thomas has commented, asking doctors to perform such searches is the equivalent of asking them to disarm an armed robber. In other words, it is a procedure that requires, he says, no medical skills. Anyone can be trained to examine a suspect in this way, in the extremely rare circumstances when it may be thought to be necessary, just as anyone can be trained to take blood from a drunken driver or to recognise drunkenness itself. These are not medical skills, and doctors should not be used to incriminate people. As the police surgeons showed in Northern Ireland, doctors must not act as agents of the state but as independent experts mindful of their duty to exercise their skills within an ethical framework.

But nevertheless, every time a police surgeon takes a blood sample from a suspected drunk driver he is acting on behalf of the executive. The blood samples have nothing to do with any medical purpose but are purely aids to the judicial process. So the doctor is already heavily compromised. Now, we may say as a society—indeed, we do say—that it is right and proper and necessary for doctors to use their expertise in this way. But we should be in no doubt that this leaves the police doctor in an extremely uncomfortable and ill-defined ethical position. This fundamental ambivalence tends to be camouflaged by the issue of consent, which acts as a protector of liberties in many cases. Thus, it is axiomatic in medical ethics that doctors do not examine patients without their consent (unless they are deemed incapable of giving it). Thus, the doctors are able to oppose forcible body searches on sound ethical grounds without having to get embroiled in resolving the ambivalent relationship between police surgeons and the state. But even so, consent does not provide a total safeguard against the danger of doctors being sucked into executive action. It might be argued that the drunk driver, for example, gives his consent to the sample being taken. Indeed, before technology largely removed the need for doctors to take blood samples, police stations were the setting for those wonderfully British scenes in which doctors would ask consent of suspects who could barely focus their eyes, let alone understand what the doctor was saying. But that consent was hardly free and informed, since even if the driver was not too far gone to understand, there was a strong element of coercion in that refusal to comply meant an automatic finding of guilt to an offence carrying effectively the same penalties.

It is, of course, the case, that taking blood from a suspect's arm would never cause the same alarm and revulsion as intimate body searches or the virginity tests that took place at

Heathrow airport until they were stopped by the government after the practice was revealed. These tests did not
involve police surgeons, but it is worth looking at the
controversy they aroused, and at the related controversy over
bone-age X-rays, since these issues further illustrated the
ever-present danger that the skills of physicians can be turned
to an administrative purpose which has nothing to do with
medicine and everything with government.

Doctors and immigration

In 1979, the *Guardian* revealed that virginity tests were being
carried out on immigrant women at Heathrow airport. This
was because under the immigration rules, bona fide fiancées
were entitled to enter Britain without going through the
lengthy entry clearance procedure, while wives would need
special clearance granted in their country of origin. Accordingly, some women about whom immigration officials had
their suspicions were referred to the port medical officers for
examination. A Delhi teacher told the paper about her own
experience but the authorities denied part of the story, in
particular saying that this teacher had not had an internal
examination. But they agreed with the central point, that
doctors were conducting medical examinations to see
whether these women were telling the truth or not. A Home
Office spokesman said:

In this case the officer referred this passenger to the port medical
officer to see whether she was, in fact, a bona fide virgin, or
fiancée. After a cursory examination, the medical officer said that
these suspicions could be removed. The medical officer concerned
has informed us that there was no internal examination and that he
very quickly and decently established that she was virgo intacto
[*sic*].

There was an immediate outcry, both in Britain and the
Indian subcontinent, and the practice was quickly forbidden
by the Home Secretary. The medical profession was no less
aghast, with the BMA condemning the practice. But the

disturbing fact was that doctors were performing these examinations apparently oblivious to their ethical—and legal—implications. These were certainly degrading practices, and any 'consent' was undoubtedly not at all free or informed, so these doctors were apparently carrying out an assault. In addition, as Mr Alex Lyon pointed out, it was against English criminal law to force anyone to incriminate themselves through a medical examination. So far from the medical profession acting as a barrier between the state and degrading treatment, as a protector of the fundamental right not to be physically violated, it had acted as an instrument of the state in carrying out repugnant procedures which had no medical purpose whatsoever.

A further example of the abuse of medical science in the interests of immigration control was provided by the bone-age X-rays. Thousands of families in the queue for permission to enter Britain were being processed through the British High Commission in Dacca, and when the identities of certain applicants came under suspicion, they were referred to a medical officer to establish their age. He sometimes decided to use bone X-rays to establish their ages, despite the level of inaccuracy the process entailed and despite the risks to the applicant. There was particular concern that pregnant women were being X-rayed, and that appropriate safeguards were not being observed. In Britain, radiologists condemned the practice as an unethical abuse of medical skills, and said that X-rays should never be used other than for diagnosis, therapy or research. In due course this practice, too, was stopped by the British government. But once again, doctors had been used for purposes far removed from healing the sick. When doctors at ports of entry screen passengers for diseases such as tuberculosis, they are furthering the medical purpose of identifying disease so that it can be treated and so that the danger to public health is obviated. But there is a significant difference between this kind of medical input to immigration control and performing tests on immigrants as part of an administrative process of law enforcement.

Prison medical officers

It is within places of confinement that the dilemmas facing doctors in their relationship with the state are perhaps at their most acute. Prisons by definition are self-contradictory places—places of punishment and rehabilitation at the same time. For the prison doctor, his role is a puzzling one. He is an independent professional, and yet he is employed by the state; his ethos is treating the sick, yet he is answerable to an institution which needs to maintain internal discipline and control. Much controversy has surrounded the Prison Medical Service, which is responsible directly to the prison department of the Home Office and thus to political control. For many years, persistent suggestions have been made that prison medicine should be incorporated into the NHS, and there have been many allegations of bad treatment and abuse of drugs within the prison medical service. It is beyond our scope in this book to investigate such allegations and arguments about the organisation of medical care in prisons. In any event, quite apart from any specific claims about drug abuse, it is clear that the essence of the prison doctor's role presents acute ethical dilemmas on its own. Not all prison doctors, of course, see it that way. For example, Dr R. Prewer wrote in 1974:

One thing is certain, and that is that medicine in its wider sense is going to play a larger part in both the treatment and control of those offenders who come into penal institutions, be they many or be they few; and in this context, it is suggested that treatment and control are merely two sides of the same coin.

There are many doctors, however, both inside and outside the prison service who view that confusion of treatment and control with considerable alarm. Indeed, so great is this alarm among some prison doctors that they are forming an association whose aim, among others, is to offer solidarity, protection and advice to those of its members who feel pressurised to use their medical skills for the purposes of control. This is because they recognise that, despite their role in a state institution where control is important, their primary allegiance is to the ethics of their profession which requires them to heal the sick and not act as a tool of the state. But since they are prison doctors, they face a real dilemma here, illustrated by the Declaration of Geneva which says: 'The health of my patient will be my first consideration. . . . A doctor shall preserve absolute secrecy on all he knows about his patient because of the confidence entrusted in him': and among other unethical practices is 'Collaboration in any form of medical service in which the doctor does not have medical independence'.

All these principles are to some extent compromised by the prison medical officer's position. The difficulties he may face were summed up in a report for the Council for Science and Society. This commented:

Ethical questions arise when doctors are called to deal with 'emergencies' wherever they occur. Is the emergency a crisis in the individual's medical condition? Or is it one of management? The distinction is often a fine one, and can present a crisis of conscience for the professional. . . . Highly authoritarian regimes are easiest to operate, and it is often these which provide the flashpoint of disturbance. So when the Governor calls on his medical officer for advice, he must often be tempted to wish for 'control by the needle', and for some good reason for medical intervention. And who can blame him, when his concern is for the greatest good for the greatest number? Who can blame him, too, when to place a man in a body belt is the only alternative means of containing his behaviour?

As one former prison governor put it:

We once had a prisoner who broke up his cell. We said he was mad, but the doctors said he was a discipline problem. So they just pumped him up with large numbers of tranquilisers. But actually there's no black and white distinction between madness and non-madness. There may be a prisoner who's basically rational, but the pressure of facing 25 years in prison may affect his rationality at times.

There is also, of course, the other side of the coin—pressure of imprisonment. These are grey areas indeed, but discussion of them barely occurs.

The trouble is that, if the prison governor is in a delicate ethical position, so too is the prison doctor—and he has precious little written guidance to help him. Indeed, the Standard Minimum Rules for the Treatment of Prisoners not only have no force of law in Britain but are positively unhelpful in places. Take, for example, the section of the rules covering the responsibility of the prison doctor towards punishment inside the prison. It says:

Punishment by close confinement or reduction of diet shall never be inflicted unless the medical officer has examined the prisoner and certified in writing that he is fit to sustain it. The same shall apply to any other punishment that may be prejudicial to the physical or mental health of a prisoner.

But this conflicts with an earlier injunction in the same guidelines: 'The medical officer shall have the care of the physical and mental health of the prisoners.' If the doctor is responsible for the prisoner's health, then it makes little sense for him to sanction punishments that may be injurious to health—indeed, the very fact that he is asked to certify the prisoner fit implies that the punishment carries such a danger to health. In Britain, one thinks particularly of the punishments of solitary confinement, sometimes for months at a time, which are imposed and which must carry a risk of damage to the prisoner's mental or physical well-being. For the medical officer to sanction such a punishment transforms him from a person who cares and heals to an arm of the state—and, moreover, implicates him in any damage to the prisoner that such a punishment may cause. In addition, this provision in the Standard Minimum Rules conflicts with the code of ethics drafted by the Council for International Organisations of the Medical Sciences. This says:

It is also a contravention of medical ethics for physicians to be in any other relationship with prisoners or detainees that is not a medical relationship in the sense that its purpose is the protection or improvement of the health of the prisoner or detainee and would be accepted as such outside the prison environment. It follows that it is a contravention of medical ethics for physicians to apply their knowledge and skills in order to assist in methods of interrogation or to certify prisoners or detainees as fit for any form of punishment that may adversely affect physical or mental health.

Prison doctors face another set of dilemmas regarding the treatment of mentally ill prisoners in their care. There are many people in prison who should not be there because they need psychiatric treatment. They are in prison because their disorder was not recognised at the time of their offence, or because no psychiatric hospital will take them, or because the Home Secretary does not want them to move. They may require compulsory treatment for their illness, but since doctors are prohibited by law from treating a prisoner against his will, the doctor is faced with a difficult problem. Does he treat the patient against his will, and so break the law, or does he observe the law and breach his ethical duty to treat illness? An example of this dilemma has been provided by the case of Peter Sutcliffe, the Yorkshire Ripper. He was sentenced to imprisonment, since the jury at his trial rejected the evidence by psychiatrists that he was suffering from paranoid schizophrenia. But it was the unanimous judgement of six psychiatrists who saw him after his arrest that he was suffering from this particular illness and should be treated in hospital. Since his condition was deteriorating, the prison medical officer at Parkhurst prison and a professor of psychiatry signed the necessary forms to have Sutcliffe transferred to a special hospital. But the transfer was delayed by the Home Secretary, whose approval is required under the Mental Health Act to decide whether such a transfer is 'expedient and in the public interest'. His refusal, for reasons which had nothing to do with medical judgement, meant that Sutcliffe had to deteriorate in prison until he was eventually transferred to hospital. So how did this place the medical officer in whose care he was? Did it not mean that, as far as this particular prisoner/patient was concerned, that doctor was more involved in containment than treatment?

Of course, the forensic psychiatrist's dilemmas do not stop outside the prison walls; on the contrary, they are just as pronounced in the special hospitals. For although these are not prisons, in name at least, since they are hospitals run by the Department of Health, they are prisons in fact, since they are designed for patients who present a danger to society and need to be locked up in conditions of maximum security. Thus they operate with twin aims of security and treatment, aims which are not always mutually compatible. As in prisons, doctors in the special hospitals are state employees and are subject to the Official Secrets Act. Once again, the Home Secretary has a role to play in that patients under restriction orders can only be released at the discretion of the Home Secretary. So situations can and do arise in which doctors are faced with patients in their hospital who are there because of a political decision that they should remain, a decision which may have rejected the medical evidence submitted by the hospital psychiatrists. In addition, there is a 'stage army' of patients who are more incompetent than ill or dangerous but remain in the special hospitals because there is nowhere else for them to go. The other side of the coin is that the special hospitals are horrifically overcrowded, as are the local prisons. But unlike the prisons, which cannot refuse to take prisoners sent to them by the courts, the special hospitals can refuse to admit patients. Many who are in need of psychiatric treatment are sent to prison, even though they need hospital treatment, because the hospitals won't take them. So doctors at the hospitals are involved in the unedifying process of refusing to treat those who need their help. This ethically dubious practice can result in another ethical dilemma for the prison doctor, who finds he is by law unable to treat a psychiatrically ill prisoner against his will. So the prisoner who is shunted between the two kinds of institution ends up getting no treatment at all.

But in fact, the dilemmas of the special hospital doctor, although more acute, are no different in kind from those of any doctor who acts under the Mental Health Act to detain a patient who is dangerous or non-treatable. In such circumstances, the doctor is acting to prevent the patient from harming society. This is obviously a laudable aim, but it does rather knock for six the pledge in the Declaration of Geneva: 'The health of my patient shall be my first consideration.'

5
SECRETS

For many doctors, the principle of confidentiality tends to produce a kind of knee-jerk reflex. Confidentiality is a sacred principle, they say, essential to the doctor–patient relationship and to be safeguarded at all costs. It is implicit in the law; it is implicit whenever a patient steps into his doctor's surgery that what passes between them will not be divulged. But this is not necessarily the case at all. Contrary to popular belief, it is not an absolute principle; in fact, the various codes of medical ethics to which the doctor may turn for guidance lay down different ground rules for preserving confidentiality. In principle it is not absolute; in practice it is under constant threat from the increasingly complex structure of society. Health care is now the product of team-work in many circumstances, so the doctor has to pool his information to a greater or lesser degree. His relationship with the NHS introduces a potentially disruptive element into his duty of confidentiality. He may wear two hats, as an occupational physician or an army doctor, for example, with correspondingly two sets of responsibility; he may be subject to more and more requests by the state to make his information available to it in the higher interests of society. The advent of computers may make it far easier for his duty of confidentiality to be thoroughly abused. This has all led to a great deal of confusion among doctors and other health professionals and administrators about what they should or should not do about their sacred vow never to reveal.*

There has been a sea-change among doctors within the last thirty years. In 1954, for example, a Dr E.C. Dawson told the Derby Medical Society in his presidential address that the British Medical Association had a clear and rigid policy:

In recent years, the policy of the Association has been that of complete secrecy under all circumstances, with a sole exception that a doctor might warn others against possible infection of venereal disease in an affected patient. In 1952 the Council of the Association, realising that other exceptional circumstances might well arise in which complete secrecy would endanger the welfare or even the lives of others, sought to modify its rigid policy. . . . This modification, after debate, was decisively beaten on the vote of the meeting.

Compare that with comments reported in *Pulse* magazine in 1980:

Dr Alistair Moulds, an Essex GP, sees the problem in a very clear-cut way. 'It is fair enough to have confidentiality as a general principle', he says, 'but when it comes to serious crime, or when there is danger of menace, that kind of confidentiality is overridden. I see myself in exactly the same position as any other member of society. I am no different just because I am a doctor.' Yet in the same article Dr Donald Irvine, secretary of the Royal College of General Practitioners, stressed the need for the patient's consent to any such disclosure. While emphasising that he would not break the law, Dr Irvine insists that the contract between the doctor and the patient 'is most precious' and that there would have to be exceptional circumstances for departing from it.

So attitudes among doctors have moved away from the old absolute certainties to a confusion of views between those who would find no difficulty in divulging information, and those who are themselves confused because they think it's wrong but they acknowledge they might. The various ethical codes themselves hardly help. The Hippocratic Oath is most commonly cited as evidence of the absolute duty of confidentiality, but is in fact ambiguous. It says: 'Whatever in connection with my professional practice, or not in connection with it, I see or hear, in the life of men which ought not to be spoken of abroad, I will not divulge as reckoning that all such should be kept secret.' Which implies that there may be confidences which the doctor decides could or should be spoken of abroad.

The modern attempt to restate the Hippocratic Oath, the Declaration of Geneva, is however unambiguous: 'A doctor shall preserve absolute secrecy on all he knows about his patients because of the confidence entrusted in him.' Yet individual countries have modified that absolute principle. The code of the American Medical Association, for example, says that a physician 'may not reveal the confidences entrusted to him in the course of medical attendance, or the deficiencies he may observe in the character of his patients, unless he is required to do so by law or unless it becomes necessary in order to protect the welfare of the individual or of the community.' While the British Medical Association, in its *Handbook of Medical Ethics*, says:

A doctor must preserve secrecy on all he knows. There are five exceptions to this general principle:
1) The patient gives consent
2) When it is undesirable on medical grounds to seek a patient's consent but it is in the patient's own interest that confidentiality should be broken
3) The doctor's overriding duty to society
4) For the purposes of medical research, when approved by a local clinical research ethical committee, or in the case of the National Cancer Registry by the Chairman of the BMA's Central Ethical Committee or his nominee
5) When the information is required by due legal process.

With so many exceptions to the rule, the question has been asked by many commentators, what is the value of the principle? Can it be an ethical principle at all when it is capable of such dilution? And what, in any event, does it mean?

Confidentiality

Why is confidentiality so important to the clinical relationship? Various writers have suggested that there are two important aspects to confidentiality—the patient's right to privacy, and the practical necessity for a condition of trust between doctor and patient. Ian E. Thompson, of the Edinburgh Medical Group Research project in Medical Ethics and Education, has written that the World Medical

Association resolutions on medical secrecy enunciate three values implicit in confidentiality—privacy, confidence and secrecy. We shall consider secrecy a little later in this chapter when we discuss access by subjects to information held about them.

Privacy is important to us because we set a great deal of store by personal autonomy, the right of individuals to control their own lives and thus to control the disclosure of information about themselves. The Lindop committee on data protection used as its central premise Professor Alan Westin's definition of data privacy: 'Privacy is the claim of individuals, groups or institutions to determine for themselves when, how and to what extent information about them is communicated to others'; as well as Professor Arthur Miller's 'the individual's ability to control the circulation of information relating to him'. Ian Thompson wrote that the 'right to privacy' was almost tautological, since without privacy there would be no such thing as a private individual. But privacy is not an absolute right, as Lindop commented:

In the use that is made of personal data, the interests of the individual and the interests of society may conflict and need to be resolved in the same way as in the context of individual liberty. With data protection, the solution must take the same form: a balance must be found between the interests of the individual and the interests of the rest of society, which include the efficient conduct of industry, commerce and administration. But as with our liberties, it is not a single point of balance which must be established. . . . It may also be settled differently in different societies, and may shift within the same society with changes, for example, in its political climate or institutional structures.

The privacy of medical information is no exception to this general rule. Patients do not have an absolute and inviolable right to confidentiality, and so ground rules have to be laid down about the scope and limits of the right to clinical privacy, the circumstances in which it can be overridden. But there are particular reasons why privacy is especially important in the doctor–patient relationship, as Thompson suggests. The first is the vulnerability of the patient. Since the patient comes to the doctor in fear, pain or need they do not meet as equals, and so the doctor is under an obligation to protect and respect the vulnerability of the patient. The second reason is that the doctor is a member of a consulting profession, consultations are by their very nature private and co-operation is based on acceptance of the doctor's special skills and knowledge. The third reason is reciprocal confidence, without which the relationship cannot get off the ground. These factors impose special obligations upon the relationship.

In addition, as the *Journal of the Royal College of General Practitioners* pointed out ten years ago, the kind of information in which doctors deal has become far more sensitive than it used to be. As understanding of human development and behaviour has increased, so medical records have become far more detailed. 'In the past, single handed practitioners could afford not to record many intimate details; nowadays it all goes down in the notes. Diagnosing alcoholism, for example, may involve detailing aberrations of behaviour or conflicts with the police or other authorities.' And as Thompson adds, some areas such as psychiatry and reproductive medicine still carry substantial risks of stigma should the patient's condition or diagnosis become known.

One of the most famous and spectacular examples of the limitations to the right of privacy was the controversy over Lord Moran's book on Sir Winston Churchill in which he revealed details of his illnesses known to him as Churchill's physician. The BMA resolved that 'the death of a patient does not absolve the doctor from his obligation of secrecy', but the *British Medical Journal* took a more rounded and confused view.

Information gained by a professional man in the course of a relationship with a client is the property of the client. The ethical rule is clear. Information so gained should not be passed on to others without the owner's consent save in certain defined circumstances. Doctors, for example, have a statutory obligation to notify certain infectious diseases. Here the interests of society outweigh those of the patient. Other instances occur in which medical men must on their own responsibility weigh their ethical duty to their patients against another but secondary duty as citizens to prevent harm from befalling others.

Whether the *BMJ* felt that the duty to inform society about the health of its former prime minister outweighed the duty of confidentiality is not actually very clear; what is clear, however, is that the *BMJ* had accepted the relative nature of the patient's right to privacy.

The second component of confidentiality, confidence, is essential to the doctor–patient relationship on two grounds—one practical, the other moral. On the practical level, the practice of medicine would be virtually impossible without it. Unless the patient has the confidence that he or she can talk freely to the doctor without fear that such personal, embarrassing or even shameful information will go any further (except perhaps to other health professionals who might be involved in the healing process) the patient might withhold information so that the consultation will be severely hampered. In addition, there is another utilitarian argument for professional confidence—not only is it in the patient's interest to be able to talk freely to a doctor, but it is in society's interests, too. If someone is suffering from syphilis or bubonic plague but is too frightened to go to the doctor because of the fear that this information will be given to another authority, they may not seek medical help and so put the community at risk. The moral argument is closely related to the practical reason for confidence, and is just as important. The patient comes and talks freely to the doctor because there is a prima facie assumption of confidentiality. He thinks that what he is saying will go no further. (The patient is unlikely to know that the principle is by no means immutable; nor is he likely to know much about his own physician's personal standard of morality, which varies from doctor to doctor and might make the patient far less sanguine about talking freely.) There is a position of mutual trust; the doctor trusts the patient to tell the truth about his condition, and the patient expects the doctor to keep his confidences. If the doctor nevertheless discloses the information to someone outside the clinical process, he is abusing that trust and behaving in a dishonest fashion. And honesty in medicine is absolutely crucial, because not only is medicine impossible without it but because dishonesty is wrong in itself. This is not to say that confidentiality has to be sacrosanct—as we have said, and as we shall show further, this is neither true in practice nor necessarily desirable. But exceptions to the rule should still mean that there should at least be a prima facie assumption of confidentiality on the part of both doctor and patient, and that patients should be consulted before that rule is broken. At the very least, they should be aware of the capacity for breaking it that already exists.

Disclosure of medical records

The number of circumstances in which medical disclosures may take place would probably astonish the majority of patients. The Lindop committee listed a few which had caused its members particular concern. For example, under the Community Health Register and Recall System health authorities collect information about births to alert those responsible for the care of the mother and baby and to provide a basis for the screening and immunisation recall systems. The standardisation of the computer systems had alarmed the Health Visitors' Association, on the grounds that information about children could be placed on computer without the parents' knowledge and there was no guarantee that governments could not use the information for other purposes. Lindop commented: 'We think the HVA's alarm was justified by the apparent nature of the system. . . . Obviously, some of the data refer to very sensitive matters which warrant extremely careful safeguards to preserve confidentiality, ranging as they do from "home conditions" to "illegitimate".'

Then there was the Hospital Activity Analysis, under which millions of records are collected and analysed. The DHSS told Lindop that its rules embodied high standards of confidentiality, privacy and security; but hospital consultants claimed that the HAA forms were usually filled in by non-medical clerks based on notes written by junior staff which were often illegible and given a low priority in the hospital's workload. As a result, many doctors were with-holding the names of their patients from these forms to protect them.

These were specific examples that had already alarmed
sufficient people to come to the notice of Lindop. But there
are many other forms of disclosure. For example, there are
statutory requirements—notification of infectious diseases,
or poisonings under the Factories Act, or provisions under
the Abortion Act, or drug addicts under the Misuse of Drugs
Act; births and deaths, information required by the Road
Traffic Acts and the reporting of serious accidents at work to
the Health and Safety Executive. Several bodies have powers
to order disclosure of personal health information—a court of
law, the Health Service Commissioner, an inquiry appointed
by the Secretary of State under the NHS Act 1977, a tribunal
under the NHS (Service Committees and Tribunal) Regulations 1974, the Health and Safety Commission, the Health
and Safety Executive and other agencies under the Health and
Safety at Work Act 1974, employment medical advisers
relating to school medical records and other information
about young people under the Health and Safety at Work Act
(although there are restrictions on the use of such information by the Health Service Commissioner and agencies under
the Health and Safety at Work Act). Then there is disclosure
to the health professionals involved in a patient's care and
treatment. There is disclosure to employers, insurance or
social security or other services—although the patient's
consent is a prerequisite for such disclosures. Information
may be revealed in the course of litigation, and health
authorities, family practitioner committees and other users of
personal health information may need to consult records
under their control and refer them to outside advisers for
certain management functions, such as investigating a
complaint, responding to a claim for compensation, investigating an allegation against a member of staff, exercising
powers of discharge under the Mental Health Act.

There is no general guidance on the use of such records in
these situations, and generally the patient's explicit consent to
use them is not sought. Sometimes disclosures are permitted
in the interests of the patient. The patient's consent might not
be sought on medical grounds, because doctors think he
shouldn't be told about his condition, but it is thought
necessary to tell the relatives. The *Handbook of Medical Ethics*, the

BMA, General Medical Council, Medical Protection Society and Medical Research Council all sanction disclosure without the patient's consent for the purposes of medical research.

Additionally, that indefinable phrase 'the public interest' is held to justify disclosure, defined variously as 'overriding duty to society' (BMA), 'duty to the community' (GMC), 'duty to the public' (Medical Protection Society), 'moral or social duty' (Royal College of Nursing). Sexually transmitted diseases must by law be treated as confidential, except for disclosure to another doctor for treatment. There is widespread agreement that medical information may be disclosed to the police in certain circumstances, but no one has yet managed to come up with a code of practice telling doctors precisely what they should or shouldn't tell the police—it is thought impossible for such a code to cover all eventualities. So it has been left to the discretion of doctors to decide whether disclosure to the police would be in the public interest, with the proviso that they must be prepared to account for their actions and face the consequences—a hardly satisfactory safeguard, since most such disclosures would not come to light. Meanwhile, the Medical Protection Society has advised that if a driver has a medical condition which makes him unsafe on the roads, the doctor should warn him to stop driving but if he disregards the warning the doctor is 'acting perfectly ethically' if he feels it is his duty to report the facts to DVLC (the Driver and Vehicle Licensing Centre). Under the Medicines Act, information about patients who have taken part in clinical trials or had suspected adverse reactions is passed, with their names, to the DHSS and the drug companies. Similarly, information on prescription forms including details about patients is passed to the Prescription Pricing Authority. And finally, none of the published guidelines refers to disclosure of personal health information to the various health professional and disciplinary bodies who may require it. In 1984 the BMA Interprofessional Working Group on Access to Personal Health Information developed a code of guidance covering many of these matters. The composition of the group and the code is set out in the Appendix.

Many of the exemptions set out above from the duty of

confidentiality would probably be welcomed by the majority of people on the grounds that they serve the public interest. But their sheer volume tends to demolish the assumption that confidentiality is an overwhelming duty which can be pushed aside only in the rarest of circumstances. They also make it rather difficult for doctors to invoke an absolute principle in order to resist further threatened encroachments by the state. True, the doctors fought a successful campaign against the government over the proposal in the Police and Criminal Evidence Bill that the police should have access to doctors' files. But it was fortunate perhaps that the Home Office did not try to call the doctors' bluff by exposing the degree to which the principle of confidentiality was already compromised.

It is hardly surprising that doctors themselves appear confused when the principle is applied with so little consistency. Take, for example, the case of Dr R.J. Browne. In 1971, the GMC threw out charges that he had improperly disclosed to the father of a girl aged 16 that she had been prescribed an oral contraceptive by the Birmingham Brook Advisory Centre. A *BMJ* editorial said that the GMC's decision reaffirmed 'the principles of medical practice that the doctor has an obligation to act in the way he judges to be in the best interests of his patient'. Yet as a barrister argued in a later edition of the *BMJ*, legally Dr Browne had no right to violate his patient's confidence, and he accused the medical profession of closing ranks. Compare that with the closing of ranks in the opposite direction, when Mrs Victoria Gillick, a Roman Catholic mother of ten children, fought to make it unlawful for a doctor to prescribe contraceptives to under-age girls without their parents' consent. The medical profession then said that, in those rare circumstances where the girl will not be persuaded to tell her parents, the doctor's duty is to respect her privacy as his patient.

Or consider the case of Mr Martin Birnstingl, a surgeon at St Bartholomew's Hospital, London. In 1979, one of Mr Birnstingl's patients, a girl of Turkish Cypriot origin, aroused the suspicions of the hospital clerk that she might not be eligible for NHS treatment. Accordingly, she telephoned the DHSS which told her that the girl was an overstayer (in other words, that she should have returned to Cyprus) and was thus not eligible for NHS care. The clerk told Mr Birnstingl about this, and mentioned that it was likely that the patient would soon be arrested and deported. Mr Birnstingl was so horrified at this that he contacted the patient himself and told her not to attend the clinic since he feared she would be arrested on the spot. He also complained about what, in his view, was a flagrant breach of medical confidentiality since any information about the patient, even her name and age, was obtained by the hospital as part of the medical process and thus not to be revealed to the DHSS. He was certain that the DHSS had passed to the Home Office sufficient information to enable the immigration authorities to arrest the girl, but this was denied by the DHSS. In any event, said Mr Birnstingl, it didn't matter what information had been passed to whom—none of it should have gone outside the hospital.

This provoked a hostile letter to the *BMJ* from Anthony Hall of the Hospital for Tropical Diseases, London. He wrote:

Under the Immigration Act of 1971, illegal immigration and overstaying are criminal offences. A doctor may break confidentiality and inform the police if he suspects the patient of a crime, in order to protect the public interest. Since illegal immigration and overstaying are criminal offences any citizens, including doctors, may give full information to the Home Office etc. Thus is it also legal for the DHSS to give the Home Office full details of an illegal immigrant in order to assist with arrest and deportation. . . . Mr Birnstingl seems obsessed with confidentiality; would he inform the police if a patient admitted to murder? Would he break confidentiality for any other crimes? . . . Would Mr Birnstingl break confidentiality to report a heroin pusher? . . . Illegal immigrants and overstayers should be allowed only one civil right and that is deportation.

Who was right, Mr Birnstingl or Dr Hall? In fact, it is not possible to say that either was right or wrong, since practice has been so confused. Mr Birnstingl was right in that he was observing the traditional view of confidentiality as an absolute, as enshrined in the Declaration of Geneva; it could moreover be said that if patients carrying tropical diseases were too frightened to go to Dr Hall because they feared he might do his duty as a citizen and report them as illegal immigrants, there would be a substantial danger to public health. But Dr Hall was quite right in saying that doctors are allowed to break confidentiality in the public interest—and whatever Mr Birnstingl's views might be, there are undoubtedly doctors who will agree that illegal immigration falls into that category, just as there are doctors who think it doesn't, but murder does, and so on. In other words, this absolute principle spells inconsistency in practice.

By no means all problems about confidentiality involve such clear-cut conflicts of interest between doctors and government. Indeed, some of the most common dilemmas arise out of the growing tendency towards teamwork in health care. This is illustrated particularly acutely in child health, where doctors work with social workers, health visitors and other professionals. It is accepted that confidentiality allows a doctor to inform another doctor about a patient's details so that the second doctor can treat that patient. In the child health teams, however, that concept is necessarily extended so that the doctor is exchanging information not just with other doctors but with other professional disciplines which may not observe the same standards of privacy. Such team-work is considered essential in the light of the various tragedies of battered children that have occurred. The Court report commented:

We have not thought it appropriate to discuss the complex issues involved in the confidentiality of clinical records. We would, however, wish to state as a matter of principle that we believe the exchange of information within and between different professions to be essential for the health care of children, and that this should not lightly be forgone on the grounds of confidentiality.

But as Dr Derek Pheby, the community medicine registrar at Wessex Regional Health Authority, has commented:

Obviously, no-one would wish to prevent professionals from different disciplines from working together to prevent such tragedies. However, with the extension of the concept of child abuse to include vaguely-defined emotional as well as physical trauma, followed by the further extension that a multidisciplinary approach is an essential part of the health care of children in general, there is a danger that confidentiality may be abused.

Dr Pheby's concern was that much of the information circulating between doctors and other professionals on the child abuse teams was judgemental rather than scientific, and thus far more difficult to disprove. In addition, this often unscientific information is gleaned second-hand. Dr Pheby comments:

At case conferences concerned with alleged cases of child abuse, it is by no means unusual for only a small minority of those present to have any direct personal knowledge of either the child or its family. The majority are therefore unable to judge for themselves the quality of the evidence on which they are basing their conclusions. Information is tossed back and forth between professionals of different disciplines who form judgments on it and pass it on with their own views appended, so that eventually a remarkably united consensus may be achieved by the multidisciplinary team, the members of which can then quote each other in corroboration of their views. However, underlying the whole edifice may be one single medical pronouncement about some behavioural phenomenon, which, being basically unscientific, can never be falsified. Thus a family or individual can be quite unfairly labelled.

A London GP, Dr William Styles, went further in an anxious letter to the *BMJ* in 1980. He wrote:

It is now common practice for doctors working in paediatric outpatient clinics to send the community medical services a copy of the letter they write to the general practitioner, and copies of hospital discharge summaries are also despatched in a similar way. This process is now so much part of the system that it is in danger of perpetuation without thought or concern for its consequences. Why is it necessary at all? These reports frequently allude to parents' mental health, and to their interpersonal relationships, living standards and past medical history—even a criminal record may be included. Confidential details such as these are being widely disseminated, without the family's permission or knowledge, to agencies not directly concerned with their care. This I believe to be a serious breach in the confidentiality that exists between parents and the doctors they consult about their children.

Dr Pheby was worried about the effect of all this upon the principle of natural justice. The labelling process, he said, was a quasi-legal one in that it could result in sanctions—taking a child into care, for example. But there was no mechanism for correcting errors at the heart of the labelling process. Professionals would have every incentive not to admit to errors, and the parents in the labelled families would not be listened to; moreover, since they were not generally given access to their children's medical records, they might not even know what allegations had been made about them.

It appears, therefore, that the area of child health is a minefield of potential abuse of confidentiality. Another area of concern is occupational health, where the physician's role is a complex one. He is a salaried employee of a company, yet must act as an independent examiner when treating individuals in the company, and at the same time as medical adviser to the enterprise that employs them. The two functions are distinct, with different priorities and duties, but the difficulty arises when they seem to overlap. For example, what does the occupational physician do when the employer says he wants to make fifty men redundant, but as he does not want to lose the fittest and retain the least fit he asks the company doctor to inform him of the fifty least fit men? What does the doctor do when he discovers that a disproportionate number of employees are suffering from some kind of industrial poisoning? Should he tell the company who they are? And if the company refuses to take any steps to eradicate the industrial poison, what should the doctor do? Or what should the doctor say if the company chairman asks him whether he knows of any medical reasons why someone, known to the doctor as a soak, should not be promoted?

Once again, there appears to be a conflict of advice to the occupational physician. The code of the Royal College of Physicians' Faculty of Occupational Medicine tends to elide the crucial question of the employer's consent to disclosure. For example, it says: 'In certain medical examinations . . . it can be inferred that the individual agrees to the disclosure of the result by submitting himself for examination.' Or further, it says that the occupational physician should report to a patient's own doctor 'any relevant facts which have a bearing on the interaction between his work and health', but 'the individual should be informed that such information is being passed on', which does not make it clear that consent has to be obtained beforehand. The BMA, on the other hand, is unambiguous. Its ethical guidance for occupational physicians states:

As in all cases where two or more doctors are concerned together, the greatest possible degree of cooperation between them is essential at all times, subject only to the consent of the individual patient concerned. . . . When he makes any findings which he believes should be made known to the employee's GP, in the employee's own interest, the occupational physician should pass them on, having first obtained the written consent of the employee.

So the BMA places all its faith in the patient's consent as a safeguard against possible abuse by the doctor's conflicts of interests. This is an attractive conclusion, but is itself subject to a major difficulty—no one has yet come up with a universally acceptable definition of consent.

What is consent?

For it to have any meaning, consent has to be informed; but what does that mean? How much information does the patient need to have before he is sufficiently informed? Can he ever, in fact, be sufficiently informed in order to consent to disclosure of information about himself, since neither he nor, in some cases, the doctor may know where that information is likely to end up? In practice, however, there is a limit to these anxieties—there has to be, otherwise the whole practice of medicine, let alone occupational medicine, could not take place at all.

One reasonable definition of informed consent, which applies more widely than simply to the disclosure of information, is as follows: The doctor explains the situation or proposal to the patient without bias and in as much detail or depth as the patient wants, so that when the patient makes his decision he does so feeling that he has the information that he wants in order to make his decision. The choice remains with the patient and consequently the patient's autonomy is maintained.

The definition is not perfect; it does not formally take into account, for example, the patient who is not bright enough to realise the potential harm of such disclosure and so doesn't ask the relevant questions. In practical terms there seems to be a clear choice of ethical principles. Do we value a person's autonomy so highly that we say he has a right to make a less than informed decision about something that could do him harm? The gut instinct of many of us would surely be to recoil from such a proposition. But if we follow through the logic of that reaction, we would have to say that the doctor should act paternalistically in those circumstances and, rather than presenting the information without bias, load it so that the patient understood the consequences of disclosure which would otherwise never have occurred to him. In so saying, we would also be admitting that informed consent, while a valuable safeguard, was nevertheless not the final protection against abuse and that in some circumstances that responsibility had to be left with the doctor—a somewhat unsatisfactory position, since the doctor would end up safeguarding the patient against a possible abuse by himself.

Whose confidences are they, anyway?

Behind the dilemmas of what Paul Sieghart has called 'two-master ethics' lies the question posed and answered by Ian Thompson: 'To put the issue into perspective, it is perhaps necessary to stop and ask, "Whose confidences are they, anyway?" In a sense the question has a simple answer: they are the patient's confidences, and that is why the doctor has no moral right to use confidential information without the consent of the patient or in the patient's interest.' Would that it were so simple. Thompson is talking about the moral right of ownership rather than any legal remedy. For if the

confidences are not the property of the doctor, they are not
the property of the patient either. They are, in fact, no one's
property. The situation is in fact extremely confused. Paul
Sieghart has rightly pointed out that, in his capacity as an
employee of the NHS, the doctor is not his own master:

under the law of master and servant, anything the servant is paid to
bring into existence, and which he brings into existence in his
employer's time or with the use of his employer's property,
belongs to the employer. So, when the doctor in the NHS hospital
makes his clinical notes in NHS time, on NHS paper (and, as likely
as not, with an NHS ball-point), both he and the patient may
believe that the information he writes down is protected by
professional confidence. But as a matter of the law of master and
servant, the piece of paper with the record made on it are the
property of the Secretary of State or his Health Authority—and, as
a matter of law, the Secretary of State and his authorised officials
are entitled to look at it, even if they are not medically qualified.
. . . Those of you who saw the Granada TV programmes on
medical ethics in 1980 were probably as astonished as I was when a
senior hospital administrator said, apparently without turning a
hair, that as a civil servant and the custodian of the hospital's
records on behalf of the Secretary of State, he was perfectly willing
to exercise the discretion vested in him to give a senior police
officer information from those clinical records if he judged that this
could assist in the detection of a serious crime. He added that, in
order not to cause unnecessary embarrassment, he would neither
invite the consent of the consultant who had made the record, nor
tell him of the disclosure. So, in the NHS today, the doctor no
longer serves his primary master, the patient, to the exclusion of all
other interests including his own, constrained only by the ethics of
the noble cause which he also serves. Today he has two masters: the
patient and the state, whose interests will often coincide but may
also sometimes conflict.

Yet this is not the whole story. The paper, pen and time
may belong to the state, and indeed the DHSS has laid claim
to medical records on that basis; but that does not mean that
the state owns the information in those records. The Lindop
committee was told by the Home Office Legal Adviser's
branch that:

Information is the knowledge conveyed to the mind by a statement of fact, and it is not therefore susceptible of ownership. Where the statement is contained in a document, or other object having physical existence, that object is capable of being owned like any other chattel; but there is no ownership in the knowledge (true or false) which the document can be used to convey.

So just as the information about patients does not belong to doctors or the state, it does not belong to the patients themselves either.

If no-one actually owns the information in the medical records, who should control them? Ultimately, it would seem clear that it should be the patient. The state may own the paper the records are written on, and the words may have been written by the doctor, but the information in the records is about the patient and since its disclosure may threaten his liberty or happiness or do him harm in some other way it seems right that disclosure should hinge around his consent wherever this is practicable.

David Kenny, the administrator of the North West Thames Regional Health Authority, argued some years ago that the administrative way to reduce the confusion in this area was to introduce the concept of custodianship:

In essence, custodianship signifies that range of responsibilities in relation to the custody of confidential information which is imposed upon and accepted by a [health care] institution as a whole. It is a general duty imposed upon all who work in an institution, no matter what professional codes govern their actions and no matter upon what basis they handle records or data, whether they generate, manipulate, transmit or simply store that data. The standard of confidentiality to be achieved within that institution would be agreed by the institution in consultation with medical and on occasions other professional interests, but the overall responsibility for ensuring that the standard was maintained would fall to the institution.

One point of Kenny's proposal was to deny doctors the right to decide on their own whether medical records should be disclosed. As he rightly pointed out, since patients give their implicit consent to disclosure of their records only to others in the health team for the purposes of the patients' clinical care, it is not proper for the doctor to pass that information on to anyone else. But despite the practice of individual doctors—for example, Dr Browne in the Brook Advisory Bureau case—medical codes do accentuate the importance of getting the patient's consent to disclosure. The BMA is clear on the issue:

Every effort should be made to enable the patient to understand the implications of releasing information, and the extent of the proposed disclosure. Beyond the necessary sharing of information with other persons concerned with the clinical care of the patient (both for any particular episode or, where essential, for the continuing care of the patient), the patient's consent must be obtained before disclosure.

In other words, just as health authorities may be the custodians of information provided by the doctor, so the doctor is the custodian of the confidences of his patient. Just as the health authority cannot disclose the medical information it holds without the doctor's knowledge and consent, so the doctor cannot decide to release that information to a third party without the patient's knowledge and consent. If that principle were adhered to, the patient's privacy would be safeguarded, even when his records are required for the purposes of medical research. Provided patients give their specific free and informed consent, there will be no problems about using their records for research. Some health authorities are now giving all patients a document telling them that information recorded in their medical notes may be entered in computer files and used in confidence for medical purposes other than their immediate care, including research. But the problem arises when it becomes inadvisable or impracticable to obtain the patient's consent. Since such research is carried out to benefit existing and future patients, this should not necessarily mean that the information must not be used—but to safeguard the patient's rights, stringent safeguards should be applied, such as the approval of the patient's doctor and a properly constituted ethical committee of the health authority.

When should the doctor tell?

Everyone agrees that this is a very difficult problem to solve. The trouble is that although many medical codes mention it, they do so simply to acknowledge that it is a difficult problem and they leave it at that. There has been no attempt prior to the work of the BMA Inter-Professional Working Group (IPWG) to work out some fundamental principles that doctors can apply when faced with this dilemma, usually caused when the doctor is asked by the police to disclose information about a patient. The result of this vacuum is that practice varies between one doctor and another depending entirely on how individual doctors perceive their duty. For the essence of the problem is that there is a conflict between the doctor's duty as a professional and his duty as a citizen. The question is, which of these duties should have precedence over the other.

The result of the present muddle is that there tend to be some circumstances in which some doctors would invoke their professional ethic as superior, and there are other circumstances in which some doctors would invoke their higher duty as a citizen. And then there are yet more circumstances where it is hard to imagine any doctor not acting as a citizen first and foremost. For example, if in the course of an examination a patient revealed that he was about to murder a prostitute and that he had already killed several, few doctors would sit back and let him walk out of their surgeries. If the police were to ask for information about a patient suspected of shoplifting, few doctors would probably agree. But if the police asked about someone suspected of murder, more doctors would probably co-operate, even though it is most likely that anyone who has committed a murder will not murder again (statistics show that the majority of murders are one-off crimes) and thus presents no danger to the population at large. So if the doctor co-operates with the police, he will not be breaching his confidentiality ethic in order to save life or prevent harm, but as an agent of the system of retributive justice. So might we not devise a code of practice which stipulated that a doctor should only co-operate in those circumstances when there

was a danger to life or limb? Unfortunately, there are two
major objections to such a formula. For a start, no doctor is
in a position to know whether such a danger is real or not. If
he is approached by the police about someone suspected of
committing the most heinous of murders, the doctor cannot
know if his patient is such a threat to the public because by
definition he is only suspected of the crimes. Similarly, even
if such a patient declared in his surgery that he was about to
go off and murder his wife, the doctor cannot know whether
he means it when he says it, or even if he means it at the time,
whether he won't change his mind the moment he steps out
of the surgery door. (The doctor might come to the
conclusion that the patient is actually deranged and needs
immediate hospital treatment, but that is quite different,
since that would be a clinical decision and not the act of a
concerned citizen.) As Paul Sieghart has commented:

Who is to decide where the common good resides? Is not that
supposed to be Parliament rather than the individual citizen?
Parliament has already laid down by law at least three occasions
when doctors are bound to inform the authorities of the State about
their patients' clinical condition: Part V of the Public Health Act
1936, s168(2) of the Road Traffic Act 1972, and sII(1) of the
Prevention of Terrorism (Temporary Provisions) Act 1976. If
Parliament does not believe that the common good requires any
more disclosures of private medical matters to the public authorities than these, why should any individual doctor's judgment of
the common good be any better?

There is another, utilitarian argument against disclosure in
such circumstances. This was brought out in what came to be
known as the Tarasoff case in the United States. In 1969,
Prosenjit Poddar killed Tatiana Tarasoff. Two months
earlier, he had confided the intention to kill her to a
psychologist, but Tatiana was not told about the danger she
was in. Her parents brought a case against the psychologist
on the grounds that he should have warned her, but although
the majority opinion in the case held that protecting people
from violent assault outweighed the duty of confidentiality, a
minority opinion disagreed. Particularly in a psycho-

therapeutic relationship, argued Justice Clark, confidentiality was essential, not only because without it effective treatment couldn't take place but because such treatment itself helps reduce violence; thus, if the effectiveness of such treatment is reduced, so too is the capacity to prevent violence.

Paul Sieghart did not consider such utilitarian arguments, yet he none the less was quite clear about a professional's duty in such circumstances.

If the doctor, as a professional, is bound by the obligation of professional secrecy, can he alone dispense himself of that obligation because another and quite unprofessional part of him, the citizen, feels an urge to serve the common good? I can assure you that in my profession—the law—that would be out of the question. If I ever had a client who told me in my chambers that he had committed a murder, or even one who told me he was about to do so—and I hasten to add that nothing of the kind has, fortunately, ever happened to me—I would be bound by my profession's ethics to resist any temptation I might feel to alert the authorities. And if I failed to resist it, though there is nothing the law could do to me, my professional bodies would take a very dim view indeed. That is the stuff of professional ethics.

What should the patient know?

The Data Protection Bill aroused the anger of civil liberties groups and the BMA because it failed to provide statutory protection for medical privacy. It allowed medical information to be passed on without the knowledge or consent of the patient or the doctor, thus allowing the transfer of medical data in secret to computer systems without the patient or the doctor knowing anything about it. Thus a hospital clerk with access to a patient's notes could transfer the information in them to the police in secret. Thus the law had not only failed to tackle the growing problem of unauthorised disclosures of medical information—it would actually have legitimised the problem in statute, had the Home Office not bowed to pressure. However, since the Data Protection Bill also provided the means for data subjects to have access to information held about them, it provoked a debate about the ethics of allowing patients to see their case notes—a debate which took doctors further down the path of patients' rights than would have been believed possible only a few years before.

Allowing patients to see their notes, or subject access as the jargon inelegantly has it, is the other side of the disclosure coin. It is all about dispelling professional secrecy, the complementary factor to individual privacy—both, as Thompson pointed out, integral components of confidentiality. Professional secrecy goes hand in hand with paternalism. It is the attitude that the doctor knows best what information the patient should have, and is out of kilter with developments that have taken place in society's attitudes to medicine and its practitioners. People are far more sceptical than they used to be about the powers of medicine and the prowess of doctors. Whereas once professional reticence might even have been reassuring, since it bolstered the image of the doctor as all-knowing and all-powerful, now it is more likely to be seen as unhelpful, hostile to the emphasis we now place on the autonomy of the individual, and may be even a cause of suspicion. And as society and medical practice have become more complex, with the growth of behavioural sciences and the development of health care team-work, with burgeoning bureaucracy and the arrival of linked computer systems, with increasing public unease about the misuse of confidential records, so the demand grew that patients should have the right to see their medical files.

A few years ago, such a demand would have been dismissed as preposterous. In 1974, Lord Denning set out the paternalist's case:

First, medical notes and records are very difficult for laymen to understand. They may easily misinterpret them. Second, the notes and records may include the medical men's fears of worse things to come which may disturb the patient greatly if they were known to him—such as giving him six months to live: or saying the doctor suspects a malignant cancer. Third, the records and notes may contain records and notes made by the patient himself or by relatives which may be embarrassing and distressing if made known. These notes and records are confidential documents. The medical man should be able to make them with the utmost frankness, and without the fear they may be disclosed beyond the profession. They should not be disclosed to other persons except when the interests of justice so require.

In 1978, the Lindop committee decided that diagnosis and prognosis should remain secret at the doctor's discretion, both because of the harm such data might do and because of their often speculative and uncertain nature. This was despite the view of the British Psychological Society, which said that it was essential for people to see computer-held information about themselves since psychological data were often unreliable and potentially harmful to the subject. But as Derek Pheby argued in his paper published in 1982, a tendency had grown up for medical records likewise to contain non-factual and possibly tendentious information. He suggested that doctors should try to avoid making value judgements when writing their notes, and claimed that '. . . the present secrecy, in the absence of other checks or balances, may have encouraged an irresponsible attitude to develop on the part of some practitioners'.

The duty to tell the truth

Most doctors would probably agree that lying to a patient is absolutely wrong and should never occur. But many of the same doctors would probably also assume that they have a right, which they would sometimes exercise, to withhold information from a patient about his condition. A distinction is therefore sometimes drawn between lying and not telling, a distinction that is at the heart of the doctor's insistence that he is entitled to withhold information from his patient. A particular example of this kind of passive deception often arises when a patient becomes terminally ill, or develops cancer. Doctors may find it difficult to handle the truth in these circumstances, and it may emerge in a manner that is unintentionally cruel—by stating the bald fact of the patient's condition without adequate preparation, or by misleading or confusing use of euphemisms. Or the doctor may simply put off the whole unpleasant business. Withholding information in such circumstances is usually justified on the grounds that it is in the patient's best interests, but this seems a dubious excuse, since studies have indicated that the majority of people would want to be told the truth if they have a terminal illness. It is more likely, perhaps, that the doctor's difficulties stem from his own failure to come to terms with death. In any event, it is possible to give patients such information gradually and with adequate preparation so that they are able to take it in and cope with it. And it is morally important that this should happen, rather than the prevarications or omissions that may be said to be 'in the patient's best interest'.

This is because failure to tell a patient the truth about himself is a species of dishonesty no less wrong than an outright lie. Philosophers disagree about whether truthfulness is an absolute principle in itself, or whether it is a distillation of other principles such as fidelity or utility. Such a discussion is beyond the scope of this book; in any event, various arguments for truthfulness apply in medical ethics and make it fundamental to the doctor–patient relationship— so much so that it is astonishing that the various codes of ethics omit it altogether. Medicine is practised on the assumption that the patient consents to treatment; but as we have said, consent is meaningless unless it is informed. And it is not possible for the patient to be informed unless he has been told the whole truth about himself. Secondly, some philosophers have said that language carries an implicit promise to tell the truth. In the context of medicine, this could be taken further to say that the privileged relationship between a doctor and patient depends on a bargain between the two, that each will tell the truth and not betray the other's trust. And not only does dishonesty violate the patient's autonomy and this contract of trust, but it has the practical effect of impairing the effectiveness of the treatment.

Truth-telling is thus vital to the practice of medicine. So it seems appropriate that the profession should at last have moved to support the presumption that patients should be able to see their medical files. In 1983, in the course of developing the code of practice set out in the Appendix, the IPWG stated: 'We support the right of patients and clients to have access to all information which is held about them on their behalf. Such access encourages openness and can improve the quality of the record by correcting factual errors and reducing misunderstandings.' However, said the group, there should not be an absolute right to unrestricted access. To prevent harm to the patient or to others, doctors would have the right to refuse access in exceptional circumstances— but then the patient would in turn have the right to challenge that decision, by seeking advice from another professional or, ultimately, in a court. No doubt there will be criticisms about that procedure, but nevertheless the principle that it enshrines, that there should be a presumption of openness rather than a presumption of secrecy, represents a sea-change in attitudes, and one in tune with the spirit of the times.

6
RESOURCE ALLOCATION

The National Health Service was set up to fulfil an ideal. If that ideal was construed as every needed service for everyone, it was unattainable then and could not become attainable in the future when technical and social advances would always outrun the increase in resources. The White Paper issued in 1944 said that 'the proposed service must be "comprehensive" in two senses—first, that it is available to all people and, second, that it covers all necessary forms of health care.' At the heart of these goals was the desire to make health services available not to those who were able to pay for them but to all who needed them regardless of their ability to pay. It would be wrong to say that this aim was not realised, since the NHS is available to all, regardless of income. But it would be equally wrong to imagine that the theoretical ideal is always translated into reality. In practice, the NHS operates through rationing, selection and hard choices made, unfortunately, with the minimum of informed public debate. The question for doctors is how far their ethical responsibilities require them to participate in these matters of social policy, since there is still a prevalent view among the medical profession that a doctor's responsibility lies towards his immediate patient and he should not be required to look further afield. Indeed, a few years ago it was common to see window stickers on cars bearing the legend: 'Keep health out of politics'. Our contention, however, is that this is impossible. The provision of health care is an intensely political subject, one in the eye of the political storm, in fact, and consequently the arguments about resources in the health service, whether there are enough of them or whether they are being directed towards the right areas, is a common feature of the political debate. Doctors

146

might say, however, that although they are part of the health service it is still not their function to argue about resources or priorities; that is the role of administrators and politicians. Such an argument is both undesirable and unrealistic. Not only is it right and proper that doctors should play a part in that wider debate, not only is their knowledge and expertise urgently needed, but they are already being forced to play it, to take the kind of decisions that they should not be taking in isolation from each other and from proper public scrutiny.

Some patients are more equal than others

Let us look in a little more detail at the evidence for the restrictions upon the first part of the White Paper's ideal, the aim to make the health service available to all people. On one level, of course, this has happened. Because the NHS is centrally funded and free at the point of use, people are not prevented from getting health care because they can't afford it. The central premise of the NHS was that health care should be available equally to everyone who needed it. But this has not happened partly because what is needed is not always demanded. There are still huge inequalities in health, as the Black report made clear in 1980, but there are also inequalities in health care. These inequalities take different forms.

There are, for example, dramatic inequalities in health care provision between different parts of the country, particularly between Scotland and England, and in England between north and south. The rate of mortality is considerably higher in the north and indeed in Scotland as compared with England. There are equally dramatic differences between the social classes and between the sexes. The Black report spelled out these variations in some detail, but it is worth picking out some examples to illustrate the extent of the problem.

It found marked differences between the mortality rates of different occupational classes. Twice as many babies of unskilled manual parents die in the first year as do babies of professional class parents. The lower social classes suffer far more from diseases of the respiratory system and other long-standing illnesses and it is also relevant that they smoke more. The extent of the problem may be illustrated by the fact that if the mortality rate of class 1 had applied to classes 4 and 5 during 1970–72 (the dates of the latest review of mortality experience) 74,000 lives of people aged under 75 would not have been lost. This estimate includes nearly 10,000 children, and 32,000 men of working age. In some ways, the health of the unskilled and semi-skilled manual classes actually deteriorated relative to the professional classes during the 1960s and 1970s. Despite the overall decline in the rate of infant mortality, the difference in rate between the combined classes 4 and 5 and the combined classes 1 and 2 actually increased. In addition, working-class people in relation to their greater need tend to under-use the health services available to them, for a variety of complicated reasons, even though their need for them may be greater than that of the professional classes who use them more in relation to their smaller need. The NHS is responsive to demand and does not seek out undisclosed need.

It might be said, with some justice, that the Black report is not about health care at all but about the wider problems of society such as poverty and social inequality. And indeed the Black report emphasises that the causes of these health inequalities are many and various. They include such class-related factors as work accidents, overcrowded housing, cigarette smoking, poverty, unemployment and deprivation in its multi-faceted forms. It makes no mention, in fact, of the part doctors should play in trying to remedy some of these injustices, concentrating instead on the responsibilities of the government to put them right. And of course that is the right primary approach even though some doctors, of their own volition, try to seek out covert need. The type and magnitude of the problems that Black raises require co-ordinated policies put into practice by the government as part of the democratic process of action and accountability. The scale of the task is way beyond the skills of the medical profession, since it involves a wide variety of other disciplines, but it is one which would be greatly facilitated by a reorientation of practice patterns, as the Royal College of General Practitioners and especially Julian Tudor Hart have proposed.

But having said that, it seems inappropriate for doctors to bury their heads in the sand. Medicine is an individual discipline, but ill-health has a variety of causes, many of them environmental—poor housing, unemployment, poverty and inadequate nutrition, smoking and alcohol. These factors should be of some concern to doctors if they want to remedy ill-health. At a local level, of course, this is seldom possible. No one is asking a doctor to lay down his or her stethoscope and march off to the housing department to insist on a new flat with an inside lavatory and hot and cold running water for Mr Bloggins (although he could try to persuade him to stop smoking). But it is possible to distinguish between the local and the national scene (or, to borrow the unlovely language of economics, between micro and macro policy-making). Indeed, it is not only possible, but it would seem entirely appropriate if doctors are to pay attention to the higher ideals of their calling—in short, their ethical duties. For the ideals that doctors have set themselves are among the very highest. The International Code of Medical Ethics pledges the doctor to consecrate his or her life to the service of humanity. And as the Black report says in its introduction:

Achieving a high standard of health among all its people represents one of the highest of society's aspirations. Present social inequalities in health in a country with substantial resources like Britain are unacceptable, and deserve so to be declared by every section of public opinion. Socially and educationally, we must encourage a broader understanding of the meaning of health and of the means of its achievement. This will include improvement in incomes as well as better housing and environmental and working conditions. Health services represent only a part, though a significant part of the task.

Echoing the nineteenth-century pioneers of social medicine, Henry Sigerist, in his book *Civilisation and Disease*, pointed out the need in highly industrialised countries for a balance between economic and social policies and health service policies in achieving high health standards: 'Poverty remains the chief cause of disease, and it is a factor which is beyond the immediate control of medicine.' But he pointed out the simultaneous importance of making medical services more effective, and added: 'Medical science is wasted unless it can be applied without reservation. We need a system of health services that reaches everybody, healthy and sick, rich and poor, and there is no reason why we should not be able to establish such a system.'

While doctors cannot shoulder the burden by themselves, it would seem appropriate for them to bring their particular skills and perspectives to these problems. Sir Douglas Black, former president of the Royal College of Physicians, was the eminent doctor who headed this committee of inquiry which was cold-shouldered by the government. It would seem worse than a pity if their medical colleagues failed to make their own voices heard in support of their conclusions, on the grounds that this was a political controversy in which they saw no part for themselves.

The dilemmas of progress

This particular controversy, however, concerns the failure of the health service to reach sections of the population. While it is just about possible for a hospital doctor to remain insulated from that argument, it is impossible for the medical profession to claim ignorance of the other major failure of the NHS—to provide all necessary forms of health care. The reason for this crisis is quite straightforward. When the National Health Service was conceived, no one foresaw the enormous advances in technology and medical science that would occur during the following decades; no one foresaw the bottomless pit of health needs in the population. No one foresaw that the combination of the two would lead to a massive drain upon the exchequer; and no one could possibly have foreseen the economic stringencies which followed the oil crisis of 1973 and which made it far more difficult for governments to fund the NHS sufficiently to meet the demands being made upon it. But long before that it was clear that there would not and could not be the numbers of trained staff, much less the money to pay for them, to provide every service which might possibly help to relieve the sick or disabled. Indeed, it is now accepted that, even if the economic situation were healthier, even if the government were more favourably disposed towards funding the NHS, there would still have to be a limit set to the amount spent on the health service; there would still have to be an amount of rationing, although far less than at present. This is because of the central paradox underlying the fulfilment of medical needs, summed up by Maxwell in this way:

The fundamental paradox of health care is that medical advances so often breed further needs and increase future requirements for care. The more infant lives are saved, the more serious becomes the threat of handicap. The further life expectancy is extended, the greater become the demands on geriatric services and long-term care facilities for the infirm and elderly. Each new advance which gives hope to another category of sufferers (heart transplant and renal dialysis are only the most obvious examples) converts a latent need into an immediate and continuing demand. . . . Every inch of ground gained is won with greater difficulty and at higher cost than the last. It is the familiar phenomenon of diminishing returns with one vital difference: no new gain, however costly, can ever be dismissed as marginal if it promises some real reduction of human suffering.

Sir George Godber, who was one of the architects of the NHS and who served as Chief Medical Officer at the Department of Health and Social Security from 1960 to 1973, wrote in 1982:

Quite a short time ago, the rhetoric of health care seemed to assume that society had a duty to provide all the health care from which each of its members could conceivably benefit. That idea might have been tenable in the middle years of this century, when technical complexity was less and costs were far below those now obtaining—though certainly no country reached that level of provision even then. Now such a goal is beyond the reach of any nation, partly through lack of means and partly because an open-ended commitment would always lead to some hypothetical, marginal benefit from care or probability in diagnosis that would offer minimal return for the effort expended. As a result, some form of rationing exists for almost everyone, either by ability to pay or by queueing for a share of limited service to which everyone has access. Excessive zeal in either diagnosis or therapy may indeed be inimical to the well-being of the individual. Iatrogenic illness or excessively distressing procedures of doubtful benefit to the patient are more common than many physicians will admit, and some diagnostic procedures have been applied to population screening with greater regard to satisfying curiosity in the observer than to improving the life prospects of the observed. The objective of providing all possible care strictly in accordance with need must remain. The compromise now must be to provide the most for the most and not everything for a few.

This kind of compromise would be needed regardless of whether a country was prospering or not, regardless of whether it supported a centrally-funded health care system or not. But there can be no doubt that this fundamental problem has been greatly exacerbated by the harsh economic climate and by the political decision to limit by law the amount that the National Health Service can spend every year. That limit is set below the amount that the health service needs to spend in order to stand still—that is, to pay for the increased demands being made upon it, according to rough computation, by increasing numbers of old people and by advances in medical technology. So the gap between people's needs and the state's ability to provide them, a gap that must always exist because of the dynamics of health care provision, grows wider and wider. And as that gap grows wider, so the clamour of complaint from health professionals increases. So great is the clamour, in fact, that it becomes difficult to sort out the various principles that have become confused. There is a cash squeeze; but there is simultaneously an attempt to introduce greater distributive justice into the health service, and the complaints from individual doctors relate to both those processes. The overall expenditure squeeze is a matter of central government policy, dictated by the requirements of the Treasury, but the reallocation of resources within the health service—the attempt at distributive justice—is policy formulated by the Department of Health, ostensibly in the overall best interests of the health service.

Whether or not that particular exercise has been a success will be discussed later. Nevertheless, it has become impossible to extricate the one process from the other when attempting to discover what is actually happening in the health service. All one hears are cries of anguish from every single specialty that there isn't enough money to do the job properly. From the health authority administrators, all one hears are cries of rage that the doctors are motivated solely by blinkered concern for their own departments and refuse to concede that anyone else is any more deserving of the limited cash that has to be spread throughout the service. In addition, say the administrators, certain specialists—particularly those practising in the high-technology, life-saving, 'glamorous' areas of medicine—are immensely powerful, since they can call up almost at will campaigns of public support, thus making it impossible for those in charge of the health authorities to resist them and thus actively preventing the equitable distribution of limited resources. It is also said that the insight of the public into the technicalities is inevitably limited; consequently they can be led to espouse a particular cause which is often presented to them by interested physicians. The cause is often presented as 'saving lives' when there may be no more than a chance of a very limited, if any, postponement of death. Here, at the level of policy-making, there seems to be a conflict of interests, one that mirrors the situation in central government. A British government is bound by the notion of collective Cabinet responsibility, so that all its members take responsibility for the decisions of government. Thus, the Secretary of State for Social Services endorses the policies formulated by the Chancellor of the Exchequer for running the economy. But at the same time the Social Services Secretary has a responsibility towards his department and the services it provides; he must fight for his department in Cabinet in the hope that within the tight constraints imposed by the Exchequer he will do better than, say, his colleague at the Department of Education. At the same time, he will be trying to persuade the Treasury (one hopes!) to make more money available generally. If he cannot, then he and his Cabinet colleagues will have to conduct the painful debate about which policy areas should get priority within the tight overall constraints—and, by definition, which other areas must lose as a result.

So it is with medicine. No one should be surprised that a doctor fights for his department or specialty in the context of his health authority's budget. Indeed, it is entirely proper he should do so. Were he not to fight his corner, he would be rightly regarded as contemptuously as the Social Services Secretary who let the Ministry of Defence run away with his share of the budget without a fight. But just as the Social Services Secretary ultimately bows to the collective wisdom of his government's objectives, and takes his share of the responsibility for those overall policy goals, so the doctor should be mindful of his responsibilities towards the immediate health community he serves—his health authority—and beyond that the wider society of which he is a part. The difficulty arises because these two sets of obligations are often in absolute conflict with each other. The doctor's first and overriding duty is towards his patients. But the corollary of that is, given that resources are finite and may be in very short supply, that it then becomes inevitable that doctor will be set against doctor in a kind of decibel auction in which the strongest voice, the one with the most muscle and power behind it, wins every time. That is hardly a responsible or fitting role for a profession which ostensibly serves the highest ideals of society. The lack of a suitable forum for reaching a rational consensus amongst the whole group of specialists is too often a feature of hospital medical staff organisation—a defect the Cogwheel reports of 1967–74 sought to remedy.

The dilemma was expressed as early as 1958 by the Medical Services Review Committee:

For the doctor the primary concern when confronted by a patient physically or mentally sick is to restore that patient to health as quickly as possible. The fact that a doctor is working in a service financed and organised by the state should not be allowed to affect this fundamental duty. On the other hand no one—least of all the doctor—can fail to be aware of the many legitimate and competing demands within the service for the money available. In theory there is no absolute ceiling on National Health Service expenditure, but in practice there will always be a limit to the amount of public money and the extent of this country's economic resources which can be devoted to this end.

There are two further considerations which should affect the medical choices. First, the clinical freedom upon which doctors always insist must now be subject to some constraints quite aside from those of finance. Medicine is not practised single-handed, but in alliance with other professionals or scientists, not always medical. The choice of therapy or diagnostic process should be in accordance with broad clinical policies to which many may contribute. Too often, there has been insufficient opportunity for the development of consensus through such means as the 'consensus development' conferences of the American National Institutes of Health. It should be the concern of the profession and the NHS equally to see that such analyses are made, promulgated and revised as necessary. Second, it should be normal practice in medicine to review results. There have been valuable studies such as the Faculty of Anaesthetists study in four regions, the review of perinatal mortality in many centres and the 32-year-old Confidential Enquiry into Maternal Deaths. But the effort is sporadic and it should be made continuous and routine.

The conflict of principles

So how should those priorities be decided, and by whom? Given that resources are finite and limited, how are they to be distributed in the fairest manner possible? What are the principles that should underlie such a distribution exercise? For unless some principles are agreed, then choices will be made and decisions taken on an *ad hoc* basis which would lack coherence and universality and create anomalies and injustice. And the choices are certainly difficult; the decisions may be painful. For example, under the strict allocation of cash limits, increases in pay awards to workers over the government's limit have to be funded from the service's fixed budget. So if doctors are awarded a pay rise that is higher than the government's public sector target they must realise that they are pocketing money that would otherwise have gone into services. (Of course, some doctors choose not to see it that way, preferring to complain that since the health service is over-administered, the extra money should be found from cuts in administration; but that is unfair to a service that is actually very economically administered, and anyway life doesn't work like that.)

Decisions between services are even harder to accept. As Campbell has asked:

Is it more important to prolong some lives by transplantation (or by the other facilities of high-technology acute medicine) or to lower infant mortality rates in the community at large? Is it more tolerable to have outmoded and inhumane institutions for the mentally retarded and the senile than to have less than adequate facilities in community health centres?

He concludes that there is no final answer to these highly charged issues, and quotes Professor Brian Abel-Smith who described the problem as one in which we are 'deep in the uncharted sea of interpersonal comparisons where there are methods of drawing maps but no agreement on what is sea, land and frontier'.

Sir George Godber has written of this difficulty:

The reactions of the professionals, especially the physicians, are apt to be exclusive in the sense that they believe that they alone are able to make informed choices. In fact, the sub-division of medicine into highly specialised compartments may make some physicians the least suitable to reach such decisions for whole populations. The natural and proper devotion of the physician to the needs of the patient in his care may make it difficult for him not to seek an excessive share of available resources for that patient, unmindful of the loss to other patients.

Choosing between treating different kinds of people in a specific situation, he said, was obviously necessary (as in a war); it was less obvious when the choice lay between services for whole populations.

It is all too easy to arouse public enthusiasm for providing treatment that is represented as life-saving, when it may actually be life-terminating for some and only briefly postponing demise for others, while offering an appreciable prolongation with improved capacity for relatively few. There is no way of presenting this dilemma in simple form, yet it is one in which there must somehow be consumer participation in policy-making.

The dilemma arises because there seems to be no way of avoiding a conflict between various desirable principles when trying to work out priorities. For example, the principle of utilitarianism is fundamental to the National Health Service, the principle of 'the greatest happiness of the greatest number'. This philosophy, the creed of Jeremy Bentham and John Stuart Mill, lies at the heart of the welfare state. To begin with, however, as Alastair Campbell points out in his book, *Moral Dilemmas in Medicine*, public health policy was based upon the need to maximise productive labour by eradicating disease through proper sanitation and the water supply. But the Beveridge report, from which sprang the National Health Service, made it clear that from then on health care, admittedly among other social supports or services, was every citizen's right. So the principle of the equal distribution of resources was laid down: if a treatment could benefit one person, it should be made equally available to everyone. But the problem is, of course, that there are not enough resources to go round. So how does society dish out what there is while remaining faithful to the guiding principles of the welfare state? For even within Sir George Godber's 'most for the most', there must be difficult choices. This dilemma is not the same as the problem of geographical variations in provision, difficult as that one is to resolve. This argument revolves around the priorities to be afforded to different services. Should we, for example, give greater priority to preventive policies rather than cures or treatments? Should we give greater priority to the treatment of some diseases or conditions rather than others, and if so, what criteria should be used to select them? Should we consider the number of people affected and the relative cost of the treatment, for example, pushing the most expensive down to the bottom of the list? Can utilitarianism provide us with the wherewithal to arrive at these difficult decisions?

Raymond Plant, of Manchester University's Department of Philosophy, has emphasised the advantages of utilitarianism as a moral weapon. He wrote that utilitarianism provided empirical decision procedures to settle apparently intractable problems about values. Decisions about whether, for example, we should spend more on education or medicine should not be taken by experts in a vacuum but by reference to what was likely to give greatest satisfaction to the majority. Such information would be gleaned through referendums, and although we don't make use of that kind of institutional machinery at present, nevertheless politicians and others who are faced with such decisions do employ some notion of the general welfare of the majority.

At a more specific level within the health services questions over the provision of resources between different forms of care and treatment, for example, between geriatric care and care for the mentally ill on the one hand and more sophisticated cardiac treatment or plastic surgery on the other, are to be settled for the utilitarian by trying to calculate which form of allocation would produce the greatest happiness or the greatest net satisfaction. Similarly with life or death decisions over the recipient of a donated organ the same principle would be invoked by the utilitarian and a calculation according to the principle would have to take into account such factors as the number of dependants a recipient had, his or her likely economic value to the community generally, and other non-clinical factors such as these.

But of course this won't do, because the utilitarian principle runs headlong into the principle of justice. As Plant goes on to point out:

Utilitarianism is a maximising criterion. It merely states that the net balance of satisfaction ought to be maximised; it does not say really anything about the distribution of satisfaction. It could be that in order to maximise the satisfaction of the majority a number of citizens in a minority might have to suffer severe deprivation. We do have some intuitive sense that resources should be allocated not merely to maximise the satisfactions of the majority but also in a way that secures social justice, perhaps in the sense that resources should be allocated to meet the needs of those who are deprived or in need even if such a distribution does not necessarily maximise the satisfactions of the majority. Of course, to recognise the claims of 'need' and 'social justice' is to bring again to social decision making highly elusive moral notions. The simplicity of utilitarianism rests upon its single principle, 'the greatest happiness', which has an empirical basis but its very simplicity may mean that it leads on occasion to distorted results in morally complex cases.

The pure utilitarian would argue that society should not spend limited money on the mentally handicapped, the physically disabled, the very old, the terminally ill, since such spending would actually deprive the greatest number of the greatest benefit. Ignoring for the time being the obvious criticism of utilitarianism, that the concept of happiness is actually extremely elusive and difficult to define, it is worth examining the reasons why the utilitarian approach won't do—why it actually fills us with revulsion to imagine that we could dispense with sections of the population. Take, for example, the mentally handicapped. For years they were contained in often inhumane conditions within closed institutions. Few knew anything about them. Oddly enough the problem only emerged with real urgency when better care had reduced early mortality, better understanding had led to the less severely handicapped remaining in, or returning to the community and when those left in institutions consisted of the most handicapped and least easily managed. Once consigned to these grim asylums, they vanished from the public gaze. Only after a succession of scandals did the public slowly become aware that not only were conditions in these places appalling, but that many within them could, with appropriate treatment and care, live relatively independent lives outside. So shocked were we as a society at the cumulative neglect of mentally handicapped people that we made them into a national priority. Now, along with other neglected specialities such as geriatrics, mental handicap receives—or is supposed to receive—a disproportionate amount of any increases in funding.

Why do we think that this is the right course to pursue? It may be argued that we cannot bear to see any frustration of human potential, because of the value we place on meaningful and contented life. That is probably part of the answer, but it cannot be the whole story since it could equally be argued that by diverting resources into mental handicap we are depriving, say, the paediatric service of sufficient special

care cots to enable all premature or sick babies to be saved
from death or handicap—the kind of handicap that puts
people into institutions. It seems that we feel most deeply a
desire for justice, to remedy the wrong we feel has been done
to a set of people whose dignity and rights have been
trampled down and ignored. Our feelings of justice extend to
minority groups in the population who are vulnerable and
unable to help themselves. Equity means not treating
everyone equally, not providing the coronary care unit with
the same proportionate increase in funds as the mental
handicap service. This is because they start from such
unequal bases. As Aristotle said: 'Injustice consists as much in
treating unequals equally as treating equals unequally.' In
other words, the treatment that people should receive
should take into account the differences that exist between
them. The coronary care unit may put up an excellent case
for a new piece of equipment to improve its treatment
capacity, but since the patients at the mental handicap
hospital down the road are living in squalor, and since the
coronary unit has always enjoyed a disproportionately large
slice of the budget, it should get less and the mental handicap
hospital should get more. Moreover, the dramatic activities
of the coronary care unit may not be as helpful to the ultimate
survival of as many patients as its proponents believe.

So the deeply felt instinct for distributive justice wins. But
this, of course, does not solve the problem—indeed, it creates
new ones. The patients at the mental handicap hospital may
enjoy an improved quality of life, but at the expense of heart
patients whose lives may literally be lost as a result because
the coronary unit hasn't got enough resources to meet even
the need of all those patients whose segregation in it might
demonstrably improve their chances of survival. Is that really
justice? Can we ever construct a satisfactory equation
between the quality of a handicapped person's life and the
right of a heart patient to have a greater chance of continuing
life at all? Having to choose in this way offends against
another deeply held principle, humanitarianism. This principle is constructed around the concept of need. The implication is that where there is suffering which requires the
services of medicine, those services should be brought out to

relieve it. It has become fashionable, however, in recent years
to decry this definition as simplistic and unworkable. Glass,
for example, has said that 'need is a useless concept' when it
comes to planning health care services. This idea was taken
up and expanded by Roy Acheson from the Department of
Community Medicine at Cambridge. He pointed out the
failing of the humanitarian viewpoint:

It is nevertheless paradoxical because although it is predicated in the
belief that all the sick should be helped, it fails to take into account
the consequence of limited resources for health care. If some of the
needy receive the very best, nothing may be left for others. We
cannot be endlessly generous and continue to be fair.

That is, indeed, the dilemma of health care provision. But
Acheson goes on to argue that as a result we should redefine
the concept of need away from the humanitarian meaning
towards a realistic approach. Need would thus be defined not
by the identification of suffering but whether we were able to
do anything about it.

If the realistic approach is adopted, it would be reasonable and
helpful if epidemiologists who set out to measure need for planning
purposes could encourage definitions of it to be framed with the
constraints determined by service equivalents. There is no justification for surveying the populations of Chad or Nicaragua for
varicose veins because although technology permits successful
treatment, resources equivalents for providing treatment are not
available in those countries.

This seems a dangerous philosophy to adopt. It may well be
that health planners have to say, we cannot meet such and
such a need because within our limited budget we prefer to
meet another need instead. But it would surely be dishonest
to say that the first need no longer existed at all, and
dangerous. Supposing economic circumstances became
rather easier and it became possible to meet both those needs
after all. If need had been redefined in the way Acheson
suggests, it would by definition no longer exist and so could
not be met—except that, of course, the suffering would still
actually exist in real life if not in the planners' definitions.

It would seem far more honest to say that the concept of humanitarianism and need is in conflict with other concepts of justice and utilitarianism. We may choose to sacrifice one or other, but we should not alter the meaning of words to conceal what is missing.

There are, of course, other pragmatic, political, arguments that could be brought to bear on this problem. Some would say, for example, that if governments put more money and effort into preventive medicine, the problem of excessive demand on the acute sector at least would be alleviated. And indeed it is undeniable that for a relatively small sum of money—certainly a fraction of the total health budget—we could greatly increase preventive policies with, no doubt, a considerable effect on disability and progressive improvement in mortality and morbidity rates. Improved immunisation programmes, better control of hypertension and a serious attempt to reduce smoking and the abuse of alcohol are the obvious examples. But such a shift in policy is not, unfortunately, taking place, nor is it about to happen. Nor is there likely to be a shift in government policy (at least in the immediate future) away from warfare to welfare. One nephrologist wrote bitterly to *The Lancet*: 'The cost of one Trident missile is about the same as our entire renal dialysis programme for one year, and one missile used in earnest would kill about a million people.' True as that may be, that doesn't help health service planners, doctors at the sharp end and those who care about all those conflicting principles to resolve now the problems of allocating resources within existing policies.

The injustice of geography

The dilemma of conflicting principles helps explain the furore over RAWP, the acronym formed by the initials of the Resource Allocation Working Party which has become synonymous with the principle of redistributing health resources around the country. This is not the same as attempting to give some services higher priority than others, although it emerged at the same time, in 1976, as the

Department of Health issued its consultative document, 'Priorities for Health and Personal Social Services in England'. These two initiatives, the priorities document and RAWP, represented the first and only attempt by the British government to introduce the principle of distributive justice into the health service—the one on the grounds that some services had been wrongfully neglected and had to catch up, and the other on the grounds that some parts of the country suffered from a far worse standard of health care than others. Those parts, incidentally, were those which needed the greatest investment in health care facilities. The north of England fared worse than the south and the rural areas fared worse in some respects than the inner cities. The health care cake had to be divided up more equitably. The principle was sound, even elevated. But there were two major flaws in the RAWP argument. One was that redistribution can only take place without tears at a time of economic growth. In a period of stagnation, or worse still, economic cutbacks, the reallocation process was bound to make existing hardships worse, which is what happened. The other flaw was that the formula itself was wrong. It failed to take into account certain crucial factors, and it failed to get to grips with the conflict between the various principles it was trying to embody. The formula itself, and the revised version which the DHSS undertook to meet some of the criticisms, is far too complex to be considered in detail here. But the central fault in the formula, and one that was not eradicated by the revision, was that it chose to rely on the standardised mortality ratio as its index of morbidity. This pays little attention to need, since there are numerous examples where health care expenditure bears little relation to the numbers of deaths. It relied on population statistics in an attempt to build in an equitable distribution of resources, but in small areas hospital services are not population based. There were, however, deeper conflicts and inconsistencies, as E.G. Knox pointed out in a paper written in 1978:

It appears upon analysis that the basic problem is an unusual one. It springs not so much from an initial failure to declare the principles upon which a distribution method was to be devised as from the declaration of too many. It was to be based jointly upon criteria of objectivity, need, equity and efficiency and one of the failings of the RAWP was to recognise and act upon the fact that these principles in practice conflict with each other.

The burden upon the doctors

Knox refers to the argument developed by John Rawls in his book *A Theory of Justice*:

Any redistribution of rights (to goods, services etc) designed for the larger purpose necessarily infringes upon the (otherwise) rights of some individuals. Rawls (1972) examines a compromise principle—that of minimising the sum of human injustices—but he recognises the need to attach subjective values to the various kinds of injustice suffered. If his analysis is accepted, then a realistic attempt at resource allocation must recognise that the criteria of efficiency (utility) and of response to need (social justice) are ultimately irreconcilable and that they may be accommodated only through the introduction of value judgments and at the expense of objectivity.

Knox argues that there is no correct solution to all of this, in the sense that one is waiting to be found, but it is a question of choosing priorities between the various principles involved, with the most glaring conflict arising between need and equity. It is this conflict which translates itself into the problems of micro-allocation—that is, the dilemmas facing the doctors caused by the mismatch between the resources they have and the need they have to meet. Doctors are subject to various levels of conflict here. There is the conflict between their duty to their patient and their responsibility towards the wider community. They cannot escape this conflict; the paediatrician who defies his health authority and forces it to allow him to buy expensive equipment will (unless he pays for it through a philanthropic donation) deprive another specialty of needed funds. But if there has to be a choice between that wider responsibility and his duty to his patients, then duty to patients must win. As Beauchamp and Childress have argued: 'The physician is not a policymaker. His or her primary responsibility is to the patient, and society has good reasons for insisting on the primary of this responsibility of personal care.' There is a strong case for saying, however, that Beauchamp and Childress take this argument too far. They say: 'Physicians are to do all they can for their patients without counting society's resources . . ..' This would appear to be a licence for irresponsibility. Doctors should pay close regard to society's resources, since they are responsible for spending them. They should as a result not only be aware of the consequences of their actions upon other health professionals and other sections of society, but they should do what they can to husband those resources. But just as a distinction should be drawn between profligacy and careful husbandry, so doctors should differentiate between careful husbandry and the failure to treat patients who might die as a result.

This latter situation is most dramatically exemplified by the crisis in renal treatment. It has been estimated that thousands of sufferers from kidney disease are dying each year whose lives would have been prolonged but for the shortage of facilities to treat them. In 1982 Mr Brian Pearmain, chairman of the National Federation of Kidney Patients' Associations, said: 'The ideal treatment capacity is thought to be 40 patients per million of population each year, but the UK achieves only 20 per million—which means that only half the number needing treatment actually get it. The rest die.' In Birmingham in that year, admissions for kidney treatment to the Queen Elizabeth Hospital were suspended because the renal unit was said to have overspent its budget by more than £100,000. It was estimated nationally that 1,700 people would die that year of kidney failure when their lives could have been prolonged had they been treated. Hospitals in Manchester and Leeds were told they could not extend their services. Dr Ram Gokal, a consultant nephrologist at Manchester Royal Infirmary, said: 'It's scandalous that this situation should be allowed to continue. We're allowing patients to die. In other countries they would live.' A conference on renal failure at East Anglia University was told that the 'ghastly' shortage of facilities was forcing doctors to play God. 'Patients were being turned away to die not for medical reasons but because they were elderly, poor, single, homeless, unintelligent and could not speak English.' A Royal College of General Practitioners' survey had found that a four-year-old had been rejected on the grounds of age and parental irresponsibility. 'However', said a consultant, 'a married man with three children earning £25,000 a year would be treated anywhere in the country.'

Renal dialysis can give an extension of life of an acceptable quality to the numbers indicated by Dr Gokal's remarks. However, the shortage of donor organs is an even greater limitation to the success of a kidney transplant programme.

There are two dimensions to this problem for doctors. Should they get into the micro-allocation business at all; and if they do, what criteria should they use to refuse treatment? A survey reported in the *Journal of Medical Ethics* in 1980 tried to face up to the second problem. Drs Parsons and Lock of the Department of Renal Medicine at King's College Hospital, London, conducted a survey among 25 British nephrologists to discover what criteria they used for rejecting kidney patients for treatment. The doctors found no absolute grounds for the rejection of any patient, but there was a consensus of opinion over which groups of patients were more difficult to accept. These were patients with severe mental illness, with infectious disease or considerable physical handicap. The doctors commented:

As long as the restrictive limitation of resources persists for this specialty, rejection of patients will continue. The United Kingdom already trails behind Europe in the treatment of older patients, with those over 65 being five times less likely to be treated here as abroad, but a universally acceptable and non-arbitrary basis for selection has not emerged. Application of selection policies based on the patient's prospective ability to repay a portion of costs via taxation is unrealistic and inhumane and moreover does not occur in other medical areas such as oncology or geriatric care. Facing up to the lack of resources available to provide the ideal form of treatment, physicians are responding by using less expensive forms such as peritoneal dialysis, continuous ambulatory peritoneal dialysis and extending home dialysis facilities to delay outright rejection.

But what criteria should doctors use for outright rejection? The editorial in the same issue of the *Journal* considers the possibilities. The medical or technical criterion, it says, is probably the most popular, where micro-allocation is based on the probability of a successful outcome. This is the most attractive option, since it involves no value judgements, but even this has its problems. It leaves unresolved the question of what is meant by success; it leaves open the question of how the doctor can know whether success is more probable in one case than another; and it does not make clear whether any probability of increased likelihood of success is morally relevant. Other criteria are even more difficult. Doctors may decide, and there is ample evidence now that such criteria are being adopted, on the basis of the patient's usefulness to society. Or they may decide on the predicted quality of the patient's life or the patient's intrinsic worth. None of these alternatives seems remotely satisfactory since they all mean that the doctor makes the decision on grounds that belong more to social engineering than to medicine. Are any of these methods more just than that used by the British gynaecologist reported in the *Journal*'s leader?

He had already selected those patients with gynaecologically urgent problems, and finding not much to choose medically between the rest, he obtained their consent to select by lot. He was subsequently criticised on radio by a medically qualified administrator for not using a better method of selection.

Shocking as the gynaecologist's approach may be, it is actually rather hard to say that his approach, which leaves it ultimately to chance to decide the patient's fate, is any more reprehensible than making value judgements about the patient's social usefulness. In addition, the merit of the gynaecologist's approach was that he had asked his patients' consent for this method of selection. At least they knew and agreed to what he was doing. As Drs Lock and Parsons indicated in their paper, one of the most worrying features of the micro-allocation business was the lack of knowledge on the part of the patients.

The disturbing feature of this enquiry is the extent to which physicians' professional expertise and position of trust is being used to translate economic and political decisions into the selection of patients, without those presenting with renal disease, their relatives or the public necessarily being aware of this process. It is highly questionable whether this is an ethical deployment of the physicians' skills, and it is preferable as de Wardener has recently stated for physicians to be overruled by the administration than for the present coercion into compliance to continue.

These troubled doctors are not alone in thinking that perhaps it is the duty of doctors in these circumstances to dig in their heels. A letter to *The Lancet* in 1982 from three doctors at Guy's Hospital, London, echoed the point. As far as they were concerned, observing financial limits and turning away kidney patients as a result was calculated to end in the early deaths of patients whose lives could have been prolonged, often for considerable periods.

Would a physician comply with a similar order not to give insulin to a patient in a diabetic coma or a surgeon with an order not to operate on a patient with carcinoma of the colon? Should a doctor ever allow a patient to die of a treatable disorder because he is ordered to do so by a representative of the state? We think not. As the patient's only advocate the doctor is bound to do everything in his power to ensure that the patient in front of him gets the treatment he needs. The effect on the district budget must remain a secondary consideration. Quite apart from betraying our clinical responsibility, acceptance of instructions such as these—implicit or explicit—can only ensure that we will continue to offer the worst service to patients in renal failure in Western Europe. Rejection of these instructions with a similar response to any alternative measures which curtail treatment of any patients in any specialty can only increase the pressure on the government to increase the allocation of national resources to health care.

These are extremely interesting points. There are two arguments here—the first, and most important, is that doctors betray their clinical responsibility by sending patients away to die. This is a stark, but no less honest for that, analysis of a situation that is not yet officially admitted. The government has not faced up to this consequence of its policies; maybe it will never do so, but it is clear that there should be an urgent public debate about these issues nevertheless. But suppose the government did take the bull by the horns, and said that it accepted that the consequence of its policies was that patients suffering from treatable diseases were going to die through lack of treatment. Suppose it went further than that, and said that as a result of the crisis in health expenditure various categories of patients were henceforth to receive no treatment—say, cancer patients or others suffering from terminal illness; or the chronic sick over the age of 65. As the Guy's doctors point out, it would be quite unacceptable for physicians to go along with such a policy. They would then clearly be in the difficult position where their ethical duties conflicted with the stated policies of the democratically elected government and would have to decide which set of duties had the stronger ethical call. Doctors are virtually in that position already. The only difference is that the dilemma has not been fully aired in public debate and the government has not admitted that this is the inevitable consequence of its policies. But for the doctor considering his ethical position, faced with these unacceptable choices he is being forced to make, the distinction does not make much practical difference. The second contention by the Guy's doctors was that by making a stand, by refusing to comply with their instructions, they might persuade the government to change its policies. This would seem a further ethical reason for refusing to comply with their health authority's instructions, although the likely success of such a course of action would be a matter for others to judge.

This discussion has dealt only with decisions which affect the time of death. That is because death is an indisputable criterion. There is a much more common and equally intractable problem of deciding how much relief, and in what form, can be given for disability. For example, a patient with arthritis of the hip can have a joint replacement and recover full activity if the surgical resources are sufficient; if they are not he can wait in pain and greatly restricted mobility for years or to the end of his life while receiving social support at even greater cost. Similarly, a patient with severe cataracts may wait half a year for surgery and receive allowances as a blind person during that period. Limitation of 'acute' hospital

services may prolong and even promote major disability for
far larger numbers of patients, for a longer time.

7
THE POLITICS OF
MEDICAL ETHICS

Medical ethics are a bargain that has to be struck between doctors and society. This book has attempted to show how difficult it may be to determine an equitable bargain. Society has changed and developed and become immeasurably more complex in the last forty years. There is now far greater stress on individualism (autonomy) and people's rights, and a corresponding hostility to authority and paternalism. At the same time, decision-making has become more bureaucratic and formalised. Once decisions would have been taken by figures of authority without question, but now there is team-work and 'consensus' and committees and complex structures. It is idle to hope to reverse this process. The scope of medicine has changed, with advances in medical science enabling doctors to prolong many more lives and cure or alleviate many more diseases. Along with environmental improvements such as safe water, mains drainage, clean air and better nutrition, this has created an expectation of better health and longer life. The standards by which health is measured are becoming more exacting all the time. Yet because the cost of all these new developments cannot be met in full by the modern state—partly because of the lack of political will to put more money into health care and partly because health care is an infinite spiral of demand, results and higher expectations—choices have to be made.

At the same time, improved standards of life have created almost an expectation of immortality. Whereas once families would have expected a number of their children to die in infancy; or would have expected adult members to die if struck down by a heart attack or stroke; or would have accepted that friends and relatives would die of tuberculosis or diphtheria—in other words, would have lived with the reality and acceptance of death—we now blot out that reality for all we are worth. Because doctors can treat heart attacks or strokes often successfully, and thus stave off death for a while, because they can save some newborn babies who would previously have died, we tend to assume that if for some reason they fail to do this the patient has been deprived of his right to cheat death altogether. If the doctor deliberately refuses to prolong such a life on the grounds that to do so would simply preserve a life that is not worth living because it would be too handicapped or in too great pain, some of us are outraged because we believe that any life has an absolute right to continue indefinitely. The fact that we shall die has been obscured, causing us to lose sight also of questions about the quality of the life we live. We shall die. This truth was more acceptable in the days before doctors were invested with the apparently God-like ability to stave off the inevitable. However, this emphasis on the right to live healthy lives has meant that we are more willing than before to reject life that does not meet the standard of perfection. We do this, for example, by terminating pregnancies where the child is believed to be handicapped.

Existing medical codes, as we have sought to demonstrate, do not deal consistently with these complexities and contradictions, partly because they are riddled by conflicting 'absolute' principles and partly because they have been outflanked by developments they do not begin to confront.

Four policies

From our analysis of these problems in the preceding chapters, we have come to the conclusion that there are four policies which can help to resolve some of the moral dilemmas in this book:

1. Tell the truth.

2. Accept responsibility for your own actions.

3. Respect the autonomy of the patient.

4. Do not exploit the discrepancy in power inherent in a professional relationship.

These policies are all related to the extent that they all stress the importance of the individual and his rights and duties, as opposed to a utilitarian or paternalist point of view. We feel that telling the truth cannot be over-estimated in its importance, both in the individual relationship between patient and doctor and in the wider sense of explaining to society what is being done in its name. Knowledge is the great safeguard against the abuse of power. The inequality of power between doctor and patient means that knowledge is the crucial component in decisions about moral dilemmas in medical practice.

In the relationship between doctor and patient, the doctor is in a position of great power, because of his knowledge and skills which can control the patient's health, happiness and life expectancy. The patient is in a dependent, vulnerable position simply by virtue of his illness and the plea for help implicit in a consultation. The doctor should be conscious of this power-inequality in the relationship and of the potential for abuse. The patient's most important safeguard is for the doctor to tell the truth—not simply never to lie, but not to withhold information or confuse or deceive the patient in any way. Only if the doctor fulfils this duty to the patient can the patient's primary right to agree to or refuse treatment be upheld, for without information there can be no consent to treatment.

Yet doctors do not always tell their patients the truth, even if they draw the line at a direct lie. The omission is often justified on paternalistic grounds, saying that in some circumstances telling a patient the truth about his or her condition would cause harm and distress. The difficulties in this area are formidable, but this attitude does beg some crucial questions. Consider, for example, a common case where the doctor may decide to withhold the truth from the patient because he or she is suffering from cancer with a poor prognosis. No one would wish to cause such a patient any more pain and distress than the condition already entails. But to withhold the truth may itself cause considerable distress.

The patient may suspect the truth but remain in an unhappy limbo of neither knowing nor not knowing. The patient may want to know the truth in order to make preparations for death. The patient may realise the truth very near to death, when it is too late to arrange personal affairs or to work through the situation with the family, leading to feelings of despair and isolation. In such circumstances, it is hardly a caring thing to withhold the truth about the patient's illness. It is correct of course, that some people would not like to know the truth at all and they should certainly not be forced to learn it, if that is the case. To do so would be cruel. But there is no excuse for failing to give a patient the chance to learn the truth if that is what is wanted. Of course this does not mean telling someone abruptly that he is dying of cancer and then packing him off home in an ambulance. Telling the truth in such circumstances clearly must not be done in a rush, or all at once; it must be handled with the utmost sensitivity, allowing the patient to dictate the pace of disclosure and ensuring that adequate time and attention is provided for proper counselling, giving the patient the means in open-ended discussions to absorb the devastating information he is being given. And if the patient indicates that he does not wish to be told any more, there the information should stop. But at least he has been given the chance to understand the most important information about his condition, that he is going to die. To deny the patient that choice is to deny his most fundamental rights of knowledge and to diminish his dignity as an individual. To offer it to him is to enhance that dignity by treating him as a person whose rights are commensurate with the doctor's duties.

To a certain extent, the reluctance of doctors to tell the truth to dying patients may be bound up with the phenomenon mentioned earlier—the blotting out of the inevitability of death from our minds. Death has been mentioned often as the great taboo of the twentieth century. Maybe the reluctance of doctors to grapple with such disclosures relates to this unconscious conspiracy of denial of the inevitable, with doctors unable to come to terms with it themselves. But it also illustrates the poor regard paid to the patient's autonomy, and the continuing emphasis on paternalism.

Here, medicine has fallen out of step with the rest of society. As we have mentioned in our first chapter, social trends have placed a heavy premium on the liberty of the individual to control his own destiny, for good or ill. Medicine, by and large, still has to catch up with that central doctrine.

Moreover, truth-telling, and its concomitant individual responsibility, are even more important than the detailed written codes illustrated in the Appendix. For it is in the nature of things that codes are broken or bypassed. Circumstances may arise which were not foreseen when they were drafted, or in which the doctor feels that his commitment to other, more important principles would be jeopardised if a code were to be slavishly obeyed. For example, as we have shown in the book, although confidentiality is considered sacrosanct by many doctors, others feel that they have to break the rule in the interests of society, when they would put the interests of the community above those of their patient. This would be a breach of the ethical guidelines in most codes, both explicit and implicit; yet who would say that the doctor who broke a confidence to protect life was acting immorally?

We have shown that doctors and other health care staff breach this allegedly sacred duty of confidentiality with remarkable frequency. The important thing is that we should know that they are doing so, that they should account for their actions. Then, if an overwhelming revulsion arises in the community against what the doctor has done, if a consensus evolves that confidences should never be broken or at least not in those circumstances, then the doctors' code of morality would be obliged to meet the expectations of society.

Accountability is the key. Many people were shocked recently by the court cases involving handicapped babies—the Alexandra case, where the court ruled that the parents had no right to refuse life-saving treatment for their handicapped child, and the trial of Dr Arthur, who was acquitted of manslaughter after ordering 'nursing care only' for a Down's Syndrome child. Some people also pointed out the apparent contradictions between the results of the two cases. But neither the shock to society, nor, possibly, the contradictory policies that were highlighted, would have occurred had these cases not sprung up in a vacuum. Before they happened, very few members of the public had the faintest idea what course of action doctors took when confronted by a situation in which parents rejected a handicapped neonate. There was no discussion about the rights and wrongs of either letting such a baby die or taking extraordinary means to preserve its life. There was no dialogue between doctors and the community about the colossal moral dilemma that had been created out of the desire, and the corresponding newly-developed ability, to save and preserve infant life.

The community, pre-Arthur and Alexandra, didn't have a clue—because it didn't want to know, and because doctors didn't want to tell it. So the inevitable happened—messy and distressing court cases, involving judges dispensing wisdom in a moral vacuum and honourable physicians at the mercy of a process which is designed not to elicit the truth but to score points in an accusatorial jousting match. Because those court cases occurred in a moral and intellectual vacuum, they were invested with enormous significance as a replacement for the kind of informed debate that simply has never occurred in this country about medical ethics—a role which the courts are unfitted to fill.

Telling the truth, in other words, needs to occur on two levels. In the relationship between doctor and patient, the truth needs to be told—on both sides—to respect individual rights, observe professional duty and above all maintain individual responsibility. The patient then becomes responsible for his own destiny; the doctor becomes accountable for what he does. He doesn't shelter behind the instruction by the Secretary of State or the prison governor or the regional administrator. He tells the truth so that he can justify what he does. And on the wider level, doctors need to tell society the often brutal truth about what they are doing. If there are inconsistencies in their actions—as might be argued, for example, when doctors perform abortions but refuse to end the life of a person suffering from senile dementia—these inconsistencies need to be made known and debated between the profession and the society it serves. We may decide that those policies are the ethics that we wish to apply, regardless of their internal inconsistency, but only after open debate can doctors claim to be acting in accordance with society's wishes. If people are ignorant and have little idea of the complexities and conflicts in the doctor's daily work, then doctors cannot claim to be acting within a general moral consensus. And not to act within such a consensus, given the nature of the decisions that doctors take daily, would be an illegitimate exercise of their considerable power.

Anthropological ethics

In this discussion, we have emphasised the importance of doctors acting in accordance with the wishes of society. It may be objected that such a consensus is impossible to obtain, since no one point of view is right. This contains an undeniable truth, and yet it is a counsel of despair. For if we truly believed that a moral consensus was impossible to obtain, then we would throw all our ethical codes out of the window and resign ourselves to moral anarchy in medicine. It is true that agreement between all sections of society on these issues would be impossible to obtain, but it is nevertheless necessary to determine the views of different groups in order that choices can be made. Often, there is little polarisation. Professor Basil Mitchell has commented:

There is still in any case in our own society a very high degree of moral consensus in spite of the talk about a 'plural society'. This is easily over-looked because attention is concentrated very naturally on the points of contention. That we should relieve pain, respect life, tell the truth, preserve confidences, give weight impartially to competing interests, these and many other principles are not in dispute. Moral philosophers may disagree as to what is their rational basis and they may be subject to different interpretations, but philosophers have to accept them as given if they are to take morality seriously at all. If I had the opportunity of preparing this paper all over again, I should try to argue that morality is based fundamentally on human needs, and that what C.S. Lewis once called the 'grand platitudes of practical reason' derive from the most obvious and inescapable of these; but that men also have needs that are less obvious, though no less important, and that our judgement about these inevitably reflects our conception of human nature.

The central point about medical ethics, however, is the most obvious one—that there is no Holy Grail, no ultimate wisdom that will unlock all these dilemmas and provide the formula with which to rank all the competing principles.

Our four statements are by no means the only tools that can be used to unlock the dilemmas of medicine. The various situations that we have discussed in the book throw up a host of other important considerations—relieving suffering, maintaining a respect for life, doing no harm, benefiting the patient, keeping confidences, promoting justice and so on—all jostling for superiority. To discover an overriding principle, or set of principles that would rank those competing demands in order of priority one would have to go to an organised religion with a consequent oversimplification of many issues. If, however, one chooses a secular path, as we have done, then one has to accept that there can be no revealed truth, no final answer that will satisfy everyone and for ever.

The archive of politics

Instead, we take the view that medical ethics are the product of society. We get the ethics we want and deserve. Unless our society were to become a theocracy, with its ethical codes dictated from a single source it will always devise ethical codes to enable it to meet its needs. Thus, just as there can never be any one ethical view which provides the ultimate answer in a pluralist, secular society, so the moral consensus evolves and changes according to the way society develops. At present, for example, as we have already said, the principle of liberty and a consequent disrespect for authority are prevalent, and have been for the last twenty years or so. It may be that before long that will change and we shall once again have a paternalistic, deferential society (indeed, some have claimed to perceive such a change already under way). If that happens, our ethical codes would shift back again; although it is our contention that medical ethics have yet to catch up fully with the present swing to liberty.

This shifting consensus comes about through continuous debate. That is why truth-telling is so important, to stimulate and inform that debate without which medical ethics simply cannot evolve. The debate consists of different viewpoints being put. The question of which viewpoint wins depends upon which group has sufficient ability or power or clout to defeat all the others. This may not be an ideal means for the ultimate truth to be revealed; but as we have already said, there is no ultimate truth, only a series of rather imperfect pragmatic compromises. And the vehicle through which such compromises are propelled into law and general acceptance is called politics. When the political debate is won, then, in due course, the idea may become a settled, agreed form of behaviour. To this extent, ethics may be called the archive of politics. Abortion is a good example of an idea that almost represented a major shift in society's moral attitudes. The Abortion Act 1967 was passed only after the most violently polarised and intense debate. While there was never any chance that the passage of such a law would have eventually mollified its most passionate opponent, the Roman Catholic Church, it did seem for a while that the majority of people were quite happy with the legislation of abortion and that its permissibility had become a settled ethical principle. But then, medical science developed and brought new controversy. The development of the use of pros-taglandins meant that late abortions were performed with an increased possibility of the baby being born alive. And as changes in medical technology made it possible to save neonates further back the gestation calendar, so the risk of live babies surviving an abortion grew and the legal baseline for infant viability began to look ever more fragile. Abortion is not a settled ethic. The controversy and the political debate continue; and will do so until a firm majority view develops.

It is in the nature of 'anthropological' ethics that no one person can settle that debate, or any other debate in medical ethics. The morality has to evolve. If readers of this book agree with our views then they achieve a collective weight.

Authority arises from informed agreement. We have tried to provide some answers to the problems we have described in the preceding chapters.

Answers

Life

Life to us is inherently precious, even 'mere' life, because it is unique. To deny its inherent value is to deny civilised standards. To squander it fecklessly would be abhorrent. But it does not follow from setting such a high price on life that it is a price that should never be paid. To say that life has an inherent value, that it is precious in itself, is not to say necessarily that it is sacrosanct and must always be preserved. We think that it is the process of living that presupposes human values, rather than the biological fact of life itself. It is more important to save the life of a potentially sentient, cognitive person than to preserve the life of someone in an indefinite vegetative coma. Different values attach to different states of being.

But at the same time, we would not agree with those who claim that 'mere' life without the attributes of personhood is of negligible value, thus enabling us to perform abortions, or experiment on foetuses fertilised *in vitro*, or kill newly born handicapped infants without a moral qualm.

This is because against the value that we set on life itself have to be measured other values and considerations. Thus, we would not sanction an abortion required because the child was the 'wrong' sex; but we would sanction an abortion where the child was likely to be born with a severe handicap, or where the mother's life or health were in danger. Ethics, to us, consists of a constant weighing up of values and principles against each other, a process in which there are relatively few, if any, absolutes. There is sometimes an inescapable conflict between the preservation of life and the alleviation of suffering, and despite our reverence for life there are circumstances when the degree of likely suffering and the impairment of the quality of that life would be such as to justify an abortion. It would also justify letting die a newborn handicapped child or an adult with no hope of a sentient, cognitive life. The difficulty arises over defining the degree of handicap or impairment that would justify such a step. But it seems to us that it is both possible and necessary to define it very narrowly. The degree of handicap or impairment must be grave. Such a move might be made only in the patient's best interests—and not in the best interests of the family or society. Thus our definition would mean that it was wrong to withhold treatment from a baby born with Down's Syndrome, since this particular disability is, in its uncomplicated form, not wholly devastating to the individual suffered but is more a severe social problem; and however much one may sympathise with the parents of such a child, or even fear for the child's future in an indifferent community, the defects of society should never be a reason for discriminating against a life.

We think that the line between killing and letting die is one that should not be crossed, however illogical this may appear to the academic moral philosopher. We believe this because there is a difference between the doctor's own view of killing and letting die. In the first process, he is actively ending someone's life; in the second, he is standing back and allowing a natural process to occur. It is true that much of medicine constitutes an interference with that natural process, giving rise to the objection that if the doctor is stalling at euthanasia he cannot escape responsibility for his actions. But if doctors cease to make that distinction they could easily become brutalised. They could no longer think of themselves as devoted wholly to the healing process but would have the taint of an executioner, to themselves, and to the patients. Yet at the same time they should not delude themselves about what they do when they withhold treatment. They then enable death to occur. This is a heavy responsibility. The outcome is the same as killing, and the doctor should not seek to pass off responsibility in the matter. This contradiction will not satisfy the philosopher's requirement to produce a logically watertight argument, but real life often fails to correspond to academic disciplines. If one takes a pragmatic view of ethics as being determined by a society to meet its needs, rather than a form of revealed truth,

then it becomes important to take account of the psychological realities of medicine as well as academic reasoning.

Research

Pragmatism also informs our conclusions about medical
research. If we were being absolute, we would have to say
that research is not justified on human subjects because it
cannot have the patient's individual interests solely at heart.
But we balance the fact against the possible benefits flowing
from well-conducted research, and conclude that a middle
ground can be found provided the patient's consent is
obtained. And once again, although completely informed
consent is probably an unrealisable ideal, it is normally
possible to obtain consent that is free and adequately
informed. It seems to us wrong to carry out experiments on
patients who are capable of providing such consent but who
are not asked. We think that despite the careful distinction
drawn in the Declaration of Helsinki between therapeutic and
non-therapeutic research, an absolute line between them is
actually impossible to draw, since therapeutic research is not
carried out simply for the benefit of the patient but for the
benefit of future patients. Thus the danger of exploitation in
therapeutic research is real. The problem can be minimised,
however, if the patient provides informed consent to such
experiments, since if the patient is made fully aware of the
likely risks and benefits, and if no penalties attach to a refusal
to take part, the danger of exploitation is removed.

The real problem arises when the patient is incapable of
providing such consent, as happens in the case of children,
prisoners and some mentally ill or handicapped people. In
such circumstances, we think that non-therapeutic research
should not take place. In the case of prisoners, even
therapeutic research should not take place not only because
free consent cannot be given in such circumstances, but also
because no one else can give that consent on the prisoner's
behalf. In the case of a child, however, its parents or
guardians do have a duty to act in the child's best interests,
and if an experimental procedure is deemed to be in that best
interest then they should clearly be able to give their
informed consent to it on the child's behalf. But it should still

be subject to rigorous scrutiny by an ethical committee, which should include lay representation, to ensure that it is the child's best interests that decide the outcome.

As far as mentally ill or handicapped people are concerned, the situation becomes even more complex. Mentally handicapped people may not be capable of informed consent, but they are nevertheless autonomous individuals with rights, just as children are. Experiments should not be performed upon such handicapped people without the consent of their parents or relatives; but even this may not be sufficient safeguard. As we have already seen, the parents' wishes for a child may be overturned by a court if it decides they are not in the child's best interests, and this is particularly the case with mentally handicapped children whose condition tends to pose a greater problem for society than for the child itself. An example of this occurred in 1976 in the case of *Re D*, when Mrs Justice Heilbron decided, against the wishes of the parents of a mentally handicapped eighteen-year-old girl and of her doctor, that the child should not be sterilised. The judge concluded in this case: '. . . the likelihood is that in later years she will be able to make her own choice where, I believe, the frustration and resentment of realising (as she would one day) what had happened could be devastating . . .'

As is the case with normal children, the courts should always be available as a last resort to decide what is best for the child or mentally handicapped individual. But clearly it would be impractical and unwise to rely on the courts for regular guidance on such issues. Yet there is a case for a further safeguard beyond the parents or guardians. As with ordinary children, the hospital's ethical committee should be able to provide such a safeguard, provided that it is a multidisciplinary committee able to take into consideration the fact that such cases often present social and not medical problems, and that such decisions often balance the good of the individual against the good of society. Doctors by themselves cannot decide what are the best interests of society, and it is unfair and unwise to expect them to shoulder such a burden. A properly constituted ethical committee would be a valuable safeguard for patients and, in the long term, for doctors themselves.

The same consideration should apply to the mentally ill. Some mentally ill people can give their consent to experimental treatment, and the law has now recognised this in some circumstances. It has also recognised the need for second opinions when doctors think experimental, hazardous or irreversible treatment is necessary. But it has not recognised that mental illness, like mental handicap, can also present grave conflicts between the good of the individual and the good of the community, conflicts which need the opinion of a wider range of disciplines than medicine. To that extent, the law has stepped in the right direction, but it still has some way to go before the requirements of patient autonomy in this area are fully met. Doctors are often highly anxious about the concept of 'medicine by committee', and of course we are not suggesting that their daily routine work should be conducted with reference all the time to a monitoring group. But research and experimentation is different, because of the greatly increased element of risk; and those who are incapable of giving their informed consent to such procedures are different again, because they are the patients who are most vulnerable to abuse. In these fairly unusual circumstances, doctors should recognise the need for added safeguards.

In general, as we have said previously, there seems a good case for introducing some direction into research since we now know that it does not bring in its wake unalloyed benefit. If we leave it as it is at present, random and without a guiding philosophy, we are before long going to find ourselves truly in a moral wilderness.

State

Truth-telling is a principle that should play a major part in tackling the problems that arise from the doctor's relationship with the state, his duty to keep confidences and his part in the national allocation of resources. Many of the problems that confront the doctor in his relations with the state revolve around the central issue—should he put the interests of society above those of his patients? Or, conversely, should he ever put the interests of his patients first when this means breaking the law in a democratic society? The answer to both questions must be, in some circumstances, Yes. The best safeguard for the community is for the doctor to tell the truth about what he has done, to be accountable for his actions. The lesson of the Nazi period for doctors was that they should never allow the state to dictate to them against their conscience. Even in a democracy—and Hitler did, after all, come to power lawfully—the doctor, like any individual citizen, should not be forced to act against his conscience. The safeguard against anarchy is that the doctor should give account of why he is resisting such instruction. Supposing, to take an extreme example in this country, doctors were required by law to conduct forcible internal searches of suspects in police stations and prisons purely to produce evidence in criminal trials. Or, to take another even more extreme example, suppose doctors in Northern Ireland were required by law to co-operate in the infliction of inhuman or degrading treatment. We have no doubt that if either of these hypothetical and unlikely circumstances were to occur, doctors would not only be acting morally properly by refusing to participate—they would be acting immorally and improperly if they did participate.

Accountability cannot be over-emphasised in the doctor's relationship with the state, and that is why the position of doctors in the prison medical service is so difficult. We have already explained some of the potential conflicts that can arise from the doctor's position inside the non-therapeutic, punitive environment of a prison. That potential becomes more dangerous when the doctor is directly employed by the state and is covered by the Official Secrets Act. That is a classic example of doctors failing to tell the truth to society— because they are actually prevented by law from doing so. And without discussing the issues that arise in prison, the dilemmas they face, the problems they have to tackle, without any kind of dialogue with the community there can be no accountability to the public at all. It is no good for doctors working in prison to take refuge behind the constitutional position that they are accountable to the Home Secretary. That's fine in theory, but in practice the Home Secretary is no more aware of what the average prison doctor

does than he is of how many arrests a particular police
constable has made in a week. For all practical purposes, that
accountability is a myth. The prison department has never
mounted anything like a convincing case against the idea of
incorporating prison doctors into the National Health
Service. Only if that were to happen would the prison
medical service begin to fulfil its bargain with the community. But whether inside prisons or outside, whether covered
by the Official Secrets Act or open to public scrutiny, doctors
should never allow themselves to participate in, or condone
in any way, torture or inhuman or degrading treatment.

Secrets

As for keeping confidences, we have shown the large number
of exceptions to the allegedly sacred rule that take place all
the time. The problem here is that the doctor's commitment
to confidentiality has been overtaken by the bureaucratisation
of his discipline and of society, and the vacuum at the heart of
it—that information about a patient actually belongs to no
one at all—has contributed to the muddle. It is surely time to
sort that muddle out. Legally, no one may have ownership of
the information, but the uses made of it must be controlled
by the patient. To think otherwise would be to deny
individual privacy, and with that, individual autonomy. The
doctor should surely be seen as the custodian of the patient's
information and the health authority must be responsible for
the standards set by the doctor. So, as David Kenny suggests,
the health authority becomes the vehicle through which
doctors may decide to make information known or not; but
those doctors should only take those decisions after consulting the patients who are the subjects of such data.

Resources

The conflict in a doctor between his commitment to his
patient and his commitment to society is particularly acute in
the allocation of National Health Service resources. There is
no way in which the doctor can actually maintain an equal
balance between the two competing demands. He must put
his individual patients first, must fight for their interests, for
that is the core of his professional duty. But that is by no

means the end of the matter. Despite this unavoidable duty, there is no need for society to suffer the highly unjust 'decibel auction' that tends to characterise the distribution of health care resources. In a civilised society, health care planning is important, to equalise facilities as far as is possible and to spend taxpayers' money consistently and wisely. It is not the function of doctors to organise that planning; it is the function of the bureaucrats and politicians who run the National Health Service. But doctors could make a far greater impact upon that process than they do at present. At the moment, the running is made by a few highly articulate and politicised doctors who realise the power of public relations and who can mobilise public opinion behind them, to the impotent fury of all the other less visible disciplines which tend to lose out as a result of this process. But the public remains startlingly ignorant about the hard choices that have to be made in allocating money, and the often harsh truths that follow a successful campaign by some high-profile specialty. They remain ignorant because no government will ever tell them; it is far too much of a political risk. And the doctors don't see it as their role to tell them. They should. Educating the public, telling the community the truth about its unrealisable expectations, about the analyses made by civil servants and administrators of different needs for health care, about the harsh options of choice between different sections of the health service; perhaps, above all, about the damage we do to ourselves through our environment and life-style, taking a lead in health prevention rather than simply sticking to the already overwhelmed cures—all this means telling the public the truth, in the widest possible sense, promoting the informed debate that is at present so conspicuously lacking and thus helping play a part in the political process of allocation, rather than settling into the role of passive instruments of policy.

What should be done

We have tried to show in this book some of the many conflicting demands and principles which make the practice of medicine so difficult, and some of the contradictions and inadequacies in the medical codes and guidelines that already exist. Many doctors, of course, are impatient with some abstract discussions because they seem so distant from the day-to-day requirements of their work. Every case is unique, they say, and ethical codes are so complex and various that it seems a futile task to try to relate practice to philosophy. They tend to be highly suspicious of any suggestion that the practice of their profession should be governed by more rules which would clutter up and fetter their individual professional judgement. We have some sympathy with that view.

There is nothing more irritating for the preoccupied professional than being preached at by people who cannot understand the practical realities behind their fine-sounding theories. But however understandable the doctors' reaction may be, it is out of tune with modern society and unless they become more adaptable and less resistant to dialogue, they will stand in grave danger of losing the confidence of the public, with disastrous consequences.

If the present rules of medical behaviour are inadequate, then we have a choice. We can either abandon any attempt to work out some kind of moral consensus, and let each individual doctor choose whichever moral rules he fancies to govern his professional behaviour; or we can struggle towards some more appropriate guidelines. *Ad hoc* decision-making is a bad idea. It leads to moral anarchy, and fails the utilitarian standard which we think should underlie medical decision-making—that the point of resolving the conflicts between principles is to achieve the best consequences for individuals within the limits set by society. Should the law be used to lay down what doctors may or may not do? We think this is inappropriate. Of course, doctors have to work within the law like everyone else; and in the last resort, it is right that if there is a conflict, say, between parents and doctors over the treatment of a handicapped baby, the courts should be the final arbiter. But the law is a notoriously blunt instrument, far too insensitive to intrude into the daily routines of medicine, far too easily and speedily overtaken by developments in science and society. Moreover, to give the law any bigger say in the subject than it has at present would be to run against the traditions of English law. Mr Justice Kirby, the former chairman of the Australian Law Reform Commission, has referred to the well-worn joke about legal systems: 'In England (and one might say Australia) everything that is not forbidden is permitted; under German law, everything that is not permitted is forbidden; in France everything which under law is forbidden is really permitted; and in Russia, everything that is permitted is really forbidden.' Kirby goes on:

> Like most jokes, this one has a point. It is at the heart of our freedoms that we live under the systems of law by which, unless the law specifically forbids particular conduct for good social reasons, the individual is free to pursue his own perceptions of right and wrong without undue interference by the state. . . . It requires only a moment's reflection to see how vital it is for the kind of diverse and individualistic societies which English-speaking people tend to enjoy.

Yet it is an irony of our present situation that unless medical ethics does provide a framework for the practice of medicine, we are going to see the law intruding more and more into this area. We have already seen a few highly unsatisfactory court cases in this domain—unsatisfactory because the courts have been pronouncing in a vacuum, making judgments that cannot reflect the opinion of society on these matters because society has not thought them through or even been offered the opportunity to discuss them. If this moral and intellectual vacuum continues, the courts will be dragged in with increasing frequency to provide, as Kirby put it 'instant solutions for acute bioethical problems'.

Kirby concludes that

> Urgent attention should be paid to the health of our democratic institutions as they are confronted by the acute moral, legal and personal dilemmas of bioethics. Inevitably, laws will be made. They may be made by judges, drawing upon their narrow experience and doing their best in the tradition of the common law. They may be made, de facto, by anonymous officials, deciding to fund, with government finance, this programme of infertility treatment but not that. They may be decided by ministers, with imperious instructions to public hospitals, groping anxiously for a

political compromise and to avoid the dangers of the single interest
political groups of which Lord Hailsham recently warned us. But
preferably, as it seems to me, they should be developed in the
democratic institution of law-making: the representative parliament, aided and encouraged by interdisciplinary bodies which take
pains in consulting a wide range of experts but the general
community as well.

Kirby's suggestion has already found a few echoes in
England. Ian Kennedy, the Director of the Centre for the
Study of Law, Medicine and Ethics, has suggested that a
body should be set up analogous to the Law Commission to
consider issues of medical ethics as and when they arise. It
would be responsible to Parliament and charged with the task
of keeping developments in medicine under constant review;
it would have a permanent secretariat, hear evidence, issue
working papers, invite comments and draft codes reflecting
the outcome of public discussions. Thus a comprehensive
code of medical ethics would gradually evolve. On such a
body would be doctors, scientists, other health professionals,
theologians and others. Precedents for this exist already
abroad—in the United States, with the President's Commission for the Study of Ethical Problems in Medicine and
Biomedical and Behavioural Research; and in Australia, with
the Australian Law Reform Commission which is grappling
with law and medical ethics.
    Codes produced by such a body would not of course be
binding in law. They would simply be statements of what
was considered to be good practice as judged by an informed
cross-section of society. Some doctors will, inevitably,
object to this idea. They will say that codes of conduct get in
the way, the medical profession is quite able to regulate its
own standards. But even they do not advocate moral
anarchy. There is a plethora of codes in existence, international agreements and, in this country, various codes issued
by individual medical disciplines. The trouble is, as we have
shown in this book, they tend to be both inadequate and
contradictory. There is therefore a need to relate them more
closely to the needs and attitudes of modern society. We have
also shown that these issues have expanded beyond the

sphere of medicine alone (if that was ever true), and it is both unfair and unwise to expect doctors by themselves to arrive at a consensus in such matters which will reflect the requirements of society.

However, someone will say that such a body is bound to sink into inertia, as is often the case with such organisations. That is a danger, but it is not a sufficient reason for failing to institute such a body in the first place.

An organisation constituted so as to engender confidence among the public and the medical profession, dealing publicly with the new bioethical dilemmas thrown up by advances in medical technology is not just a good idea—it is necessary. Otherwise society will eventually wake up and see that medical ethics have been left behind by progress. There is then a serious danger of an over-reaction with inappropriate demands that something is done about curbing practices without any rational discussion of their value to the community. Kirby has commented: '. . . it will be the judgement of history that the scientists of our generation brought forth most remarkable developments of human ingenuity—but the lawyers, philosophers, theologians and lawmakers proved incompetent to keep pace.'

We have to develop a better mechanism in our society through which we can discuss these momentous issues and arrive at a democratic agreement on how we should behave according to our medical needs and the measures we have developed to satisfy them—an agreement about the philosophy of medicine, and what kind of society it serves.

APPENDIX:
ETHICAL CODES

The Hippocratic Oath (5th century BC)

It is not certain that the Hippocratic Oath was written by Hippocrates but it was probably written during his lifetime. The earliest surviving references to this Oath date from the first century AD. These suggested that the Oath was seen as an ideal rather than a norm and it was not until the 4th Century AD that it was an obligatory requirement for a doctor to take the Oath before practising.

The Hippocratic Oath

I swear by Apollo Physician and Asclepius and Hygieia and Panaceia and all the gods and goddesses, making them my witnesses, that I will fulfil according to my ability and judgement this oath and this covenant:

To hold him who has taught me this art as equal to my parents and to live my life in partnership with him, and if he is in need of money to give him a share of mine, and to regard his offspring as equal to my brothers in male lineage and to teach them this art—if they desire to learn it—without fee and covenant; to give a share of precepts and oral instruction and all the other learning to my sons and to the sons of him who has instructed me and to pupils who have signed the covenant and have taken an oath according to the medical law, but to no one else.

I will apply dietetic measures for the benefit of the sick according to my ability and judgment; I will keep them from harm and injustice.

I will neither give a deadly drug to anybody if asked for it, nor will I make a suggestion to this effect. Similarly I will not give to a woman an abortive remedy. In purity and holiness I will guard my life and my art.

I will not use the knife, not even on sufferers from stone, but will withdraw in favor of such men as are engaged in this work.

Whatever houses I may visit, I will come for the benefit of the sick, remaining free of all intentional injustice, of all mischief and in particular of sexual relations with both female and male persons, be they free or slaves.

What I may see or hear in the course of the treatment in regard to the life of men, which on no account one must spread abroad, I will keep to myself holding such things shameful to be spoken about.

If I fulfil this oath and do not violate it, may it be granted to me to enjoy life and art, being honored with fame among all men for all time to come; if I transgress it and swear falsely, may the opposite of all this be my lot.

Inter-professional Working Group Code of Confidentiality of Personal Health Data

Member organisations:

British Medical Association; Royal College of Nursing; Royal College of Midwives; Health Visitors Association; Council for Professions Supplementary to Medicine; British Association of Social Workers; British Dental Association; British Psychological Society.

Preliminary
1. In this Code
    1. 'disclosure' includes allowing access to personal health data;
    2. 'third party' means a person who is not an employee or member of the health authority concerned;
    3. 'personal health data' means identifiable personal data relating to the physical or mental health of any person;
    4. 'health care' means the care of a person's physical or mental health and includes the provision by a health authority of services forming part of the health service;

5. 'patient' means a person to whom a health authority provides health care;
6. 'professionally qualified person' means:
(a) a person who is registered under the Professions Supplementary to Medicine Act 1960, the Nurses, Midwives and Health visitors Act 1979, the Medical Act 1983 or the Dentists Act 1984;
(b) a person employed as a clinical psychologist by a health authority or a special hospital;
(c) an approved social worker within the meaning of the Mental Health Act 1983.

2. This Code sets out the principles which health authorities must observe about disclosures to employees or members of the authority, or to third parties, of [automatically processed] personal health data relating to any person which are held by the authority in connection with the provision of health care to a patient.

Fundamental Principles

3. Subject only to the exceptions in paragraph 4 below, the following fundamental principles must be observed in order to preserve the confidentiality of personal health data held by a health authority:
(a) a health authority holds information about a patient only for the purpose of health care, and a patient about whom personal health data are held by a health authority has a right to have such data kept confidential and not disclosed to third parties without his consent (either expressly or by necessary implication) and health authorities have a duty to respect that right;
(b) professionally qualified persons employed by a health authority have professional obligations to keep personal health data confidential and to ensure that they are disclosed only to those who need them for the health care of the patient;
(c) such professionally qualified persons entrust personal health data to health authorities only on the understanding that the patient's right to confidentiality and their corresponding professional obligations will be respected,

and health authorities have a duty to see that this is done;
(d) a patient about whom personal health data are held by
a health authority has a right not to have such data
disclosed without his consent to employees or members
of that authority for any purpose other than his health
care, and health authorities have a duty to respect that
right;
(e) personal health data relating to a person other than
the patient which are held in connection with the health
care of that patient must not be disclosed to third parties
or to employees or members of the health authority, even
with the consent of that patient, for any purpose other
than the health care of that patient.

Accordingly, unless the patient has given his consent,
personal health data relating to him or, even with his
consent, any such data relating to any other person which are
held in connection with the health care of that patient must
not be disclosed to anyone for any purpose other than the
health care of that patient.

Exceptions

4. The only exceptions to the application of the fundamental principles set out in paragraph 3 above are:
(a) where the disclosure is required (and not merely
permitted) by or under a statute;
(b) where the disclosure is ordered by a court of law or
by a person or body empowered by or under a statute to
require disclosure;
(c) where the disclosure is necessary for the proper
investigation of a complaint or untoward incident, or for
some other essential management function;
(d) where the disclosure is authorised by an appropriate
ethical committee for the purpose of health research,
provided that there are appropriate safeguards to ensure
that no damage or distress will be caused to the subject of
the data and that his anonymity in published results is
secured;
(e) where the disclosure is necessary for the prevention,
detection or prosecution of a crime which is so serious

that the public interest must prevail over the right to confidentiality;

(f) where the disclosure is necessary to safeguard national security;

(g) where the disclosure is necessary to prevent a serious risk to public health.

In cases described in items (e), (f) and (g) above, the decision whether to make a disclosure must always remain with the professionally qualified person employed by the health authority who is responsible at the time the request is made for the particular aspect of the patient's care. Exceptionally in an urgent case, if that person is absent or, in a case to which item (e) or (f) applies, is himself the subject of the investigation, a professionally qualified person employed by the health authority must be authorised to make it in his place.

5. Appropriate steps must be taken to ensure that the data disclosed will not be used for any purpose other than that for which the disclosure is made.

Management Arrangements

6. Health authorities must establish, in consultation with representatives of all relevant professionally qualified persons, procedures which will ensure that all disclosures of personal health data are made in accordance with the foregoing paragraphs, and in particular:

(a) who is the person to whom all requests for exceptional disclosures specified in paragraph 4 above must be made or referred;

(b) who is the professionally qualified person normally responsible, in relation to personal health data held for the purposes of each aspect of the patient's health care, for deciding whether or not to disclose in the cases described in paragraph 4(e), (f) and (g) above;

(c) who is the professionally qualified person authorised to decide on disclosure exceptionally in an urgent case, if the person normally responsible is absent or is himself the subject of the investigation;

(d) what safeguards are required to ensure that the data will be used only for the purpose for which they are disclosed;

(e) that records will be kept of all exceptional disclosures specified in paragraph 4 above.

7. Health authorities must make arrangements to ensure that personal health data held in connection with a patient are made available, subject to paragraph 4 above, only to employees or members of the authority who need them for his health care.

8. Health authorities must ensure that all employees and members, and not only those directly concerned, are aware of this Code and of the management arrangements made to implement it. Authorities must also ensure that the terms and conditions of employment of all their employees contain appropriate provisions prohibiting breaches of confidentiality about personal health data and enable disciplinary or dismissal procedures to be invoked if such breaches occur. Where services are contracted out, health authorities must ensure that the contracts specify arrangements to ensure that confidentiality of personal health data is maintained.

9. Health authorities must ensure that their management arrangements for implementing this Code are formally adopted at meetings open to the public and are regularly reviewed in consultation with representatives of all relevant professionally qualified persons.

10. Health authorities must publish, at least once a year, statistics of the number and nature of the exceptional disclosures made in accordance with the provisions of paragraph 4 above.

Confidentiality of Personal Health Data: Notes to Code

Introduction

1. The Code sets out the principles which health authorities must observe about the disclosure to employees or members

of the authority or to third parties of identifiable personal health data held by them for the purpose of providing health care. These Notes are intended to assist in implementing the Code.

Fundamental Principles

2. It is a fundamental principle of health care that all identifiable personal health data should be used only for the health care of the patient in respect of whom they have been acquired and should not be disclosed without his consent (but see also paragraph 3 below) to third parties who do not need them for a particular aspect of that care. To that principle there are certain strictly limited exceptions where the law or the public interest may override the patient's right to confidentiality. However, such cases will be exceptional. Health authorities must therefore ensure that personal health data are never disclosed without the patient's consent to third parties, otherwise than for a particular aspect of his health care, unless the Code specifically allows this. In most of the cases where it does, the decision whether to disclose will still rest with the responsible health professional. Certain statutes or regulations may preclude disclosure or impose additional restrictions, for example, the National Health Service (Venereal Disease) Regulations 1974 (SI 1974/29). Nothing in the Code or these Notes can be taken as overriding such legal restrictions on disclosure.

3. Health data needed to care for a patient will normally be obtained by or for health professionals, who will be under a professional obligation to respect the confidence under which they were obtained and who entrust the data to the health authority which employs them only on the understanding that this confidence will be respected. Health data needed to care for a patient usually relate to the patient himself, but they may sometimes relate to someone connected with him. The subject of the data is, therefore, usually but not always the patient. Where a person other than the patient is the data subject he will have his own right to have the data kept confidential.

Exceptions

4. (a) *Where the disclosure is required by or under a statute*
Listed in Annex A to these Notes are a number of examples of statutes which require certain disclosures to be made. Where there is such a requirement, health authorities must disclose and need not obtain the consent either of the subject or of the responsible health professional, although they should notify those persons about the disclosures where that is reasonably practicable. But it must be clearly understood that this exception only applies where the statute *requires* such a disclosure to be made, and does not merely permit it. Certain agencies such as those listed in Annex B have a statutory right to require the supply of information which could include personal health data. Health authorities are not required to obtain consent in order to comply with any direction to supply data to such agencies. Again, though, they should notify the subject and the responsible health professional where reasonably practicable.

(b) *Where the disclosure is ordered by a court of law or by a person or body empowered by or under a statute to require disclosure*
The courts and a number of tribunals and persons appointed to hold inquiries have power to require that information, which may be relevant to matters within their jurisdiction, should be disclosed. A list of some of the statutory provisions (in addition to the inherent jurisdiction of the courts under the common law) enabling disclosures to be ordered for the purpose of such matters is given in Annex C. Where a court or tribunal so orders, health authorities must disclose strictly in the terms of that order. They need not formally obtain the consent of the subject or of the responsible health professional, although they should give those persons prompt notice of the order so that they will have an opportunity to apply to the court or tribunal to have it set aside if they so wish.

(c) *Essential management functions*
Proper management by a health authority may necessi-
tate access to personal health data, for example, where a
complaint has been made against the authority or
individual health professionals, or where an untoward
incident has been reported (examples of essential management functions are at Annex D). Here again, neither
the consent of the subject nor of the responsible health
professional is required. However, all such cases must be
scrutinised by a senior member of staff to ensure that the
disclosure without such consent is essential and not
merely convenient, and that the data disclosed will not be
used for any other purpose.

(d) *Health research*
Research into health or disease may benefit existing or
future patients or lead to improvements in public health
generally. Access to personal health data by researchers
should therefore not be unnecessarily hampered, but
there must be appropriate safeguards. Although the
general rule is that the subject's consent must be obtained
for any disclosure of personal health data, in the case of
some kinds of health research this may often not be
reasonably practicable or could be against the subject's
own interests. In such cases, disclosure should only be
allowed after an appropriate ethical committee (which
should include lay members and representatives from the
research community and from other health professions as
well as medicine and dentistry) has satisfied itself that a
sufficient case for dispensing with the subject's consent
has been made out and has approved the proposals.
However, any objection which the subject may have
made known in advance must be respected. Before
giving its approval, the committee must obtain formal
undertakings that:

— whenever practicable consent to use the relevant
   personal health data will be obtained from the health
   professional originally responsible for that aspect of
   the patient's health care or his successor, or, if there is

none, a health professional designated by the health
authority;

— no approach will be made to a subject about whom
data have been disclosed without the consent of the
professional currently responsible for the relevant
aspect of his health care and/or his general practitioner;

— the personal health data available to the research team
will not be disclosed to anyone outside it and will be
adequately secured against unauthorised access;

— no subject will be identifiable from any published
results;

— all personal health data obtained for the purpose of the
research will be destroyed when they are no longer
required for that purpose.

Health authorities must make arrangements to ensure
that the above procedure for the approval of research
proposals is carried out. They should also try to make
their patients generally aware that, in their own interests
and those of the public, details from their health records
may be disclosed for the purposes of bona fide research
into health and disease and for the better provision of
health services, subject to the above safeguards. Health
authorities should encourage general understanding of
the importance of the use of such records for research.

(e) *The prevention, detection and prosecution of crime*
The disclosure of personal health data may exceptionally
be justified if it can help to prevent or detect the
commission of a serious crime or bring the perpetrator of
such a crime to justice. Before such a disclosure is made,
at least the following conditions must be satisfied:

— the crime must be sufficiently serious for the public
interest to prevail (section [109] of the Police and

Criminal Evidence Act 1984 may provide a guide to this but must not be treated as either conclusive or exhaustive);

— it must be established that, without the disclosure, the task of preventing or detecting the crime would be seriously prejudiced or delayed;

— satisfactory undertakings must be obtained that the personal health data disclosed will not be used for any other purpose and will be destroyed if the subject is not prosecuted or is discharged or acquitted.

Such disclosures require the consent of the health professional responsible for the relevant aspect of the patient's health care at the time of the request.

(f) *Safeguarding national security*
Exceptionally, it may be necessary to disclose personal health data where the interests of national security require it. The consent of the health professional responsible for the relevant aspect of the patient's health care at the time is required for such a disclosure. The health professional must be satisfied that national security is involved and that disclosure is necessary to safeguard security interests. For this purpose, a certificate signed personally by a Cabinet Minister or by the Attorney General or the Lord Advocate under section 27 of the Data Protection Act 1984 that disclosure is (or was) required to safeguard national security may be treated as conclusive.

(g) *The interests of public health*
It may be necessary to disclose personal health data in order to prevent serious risks to public health, for example, in the prevention and control of communicable diseases beyond the notifiable infectious diseases covered by the public health legislation or through the monitoring of adverse reactions to drugs. Disclosure for these purposes should only be made with the consent of the health professional responsible for that aspect of the

patient's health care and with appropriate safeguards to ensure that the data will not be used for any other purpose.

Management Arrangements and Publicity

5. Clear procedures as to the circumstances in which and the purposes for which disclosures may be made will be needed to ensure that the requirements of the Code are observed and to reflect the general duty on all employees to respect the confidentiality of personal health data. These should be established by the health authority, in consultation with representatives of all its professionally qualified staff, adopted formally at a meeting open to the public and kept under regular review. Where the Code requires consent to a disclosure by the health professional responsible for a particular aspect of the patient's health care, agreed procedures should include arrangements for dealing with urgent requests and for any delegation (eg from a consultant to an SHO) or substitution (eg where the responsible health professional is himself the subject of the investigation).

6. If the agreed procedures are to be understood and operated by the staff concerned, they need to be simple and unambiguous. Circumstances in which a speedy response is required may arise, and staff will need to be aware of the procedures which will then need to be carried out.

7. The duty of confidentiality should be reflected in the terms and conditions of employment of all the authority's employees and subject to disciplinary sanctions, including dismissal. Health authorities should also provide training for all staff on the maintenance of confidentiality.

8. Where health authorities contract with outside firms for the supply of services to them or direct to patients, they must ensure that the contracts include adequate terms for the protection of the confidentiality of personal health data.

9. It is also important for maintaining public confidence in the confidentiality of health records that the working of the

prodedures is publicly monitored. Publishing statistics of disclosures in the excepted categories at least once a year should help to achieve this.

Annex A: Examples of Disclosures Required by Statute

a.   *Notification of Infectious Diseases*
     The Public Health Act 1936
     The Public Health Act 1961
   ★ The Health Services and Public Health Act 1968
     The Public Health (Infectious Diseases) Regs 1968 (SI 1968 No. 1366)
   ★ The Public Health (Fees for Notification of Infectious Diseases) Order 1968 (SI 1968 No. 1365)
     The Public Health (Infectious Diseases) (Amendment) Regs 1969 (SI 1969 No. 844)
     The Public Health (Infectious Diseases) (Amendment) Regs 1974 (SI 1974 No. 274)
     The Public Health (Infectious Diseases) (Amendment) Regs 1976 (SI 1976 No. 1226)
     The Public Health (Infectious Diseases) (Amendment) (No. 2) Regs 1976 (SI 1976 No. 1955)
   ★ Amended by HASSASSA Act 1983 Section 26
b.   *Notifications of Poisonings and Other Serious Accidents at Work*
   ★ The Factories Act 1961, Section 82
     The Health and Safety at Work etc Act 1974
   ★ The Notification of Accidents and Dangerous Occurrences Regs 1980 (SI 1980 No. 804)
   ★ Currently being revised by the Health and Safety Executive
c.   *Notifications of Abortions*
     Abortion Act 1967, Section 2
     The Abortion Regs 1968 (SI 1968 No. 390)
     The Abortion (Amendment) Regs 1969 (SI 1969 No 636)
     The Abortion (Amendment) Regs 1976 (SI 1976 No 15)
     The Abortion (Amendment) Regs 1980 (SI 1980 No 1724)
d.   *Notification of Drug Addicts*
     Misuse of Drugs Act 1971, Section 10
     Misuse of Drugs (Notification of and Supply of Addicts) Regs 1973 (SI 1973 No 799)
e.   *Notifications of Births and Deaths*
     The National Health Service Act 1977, Section 124
     The National Health Service (Notification of Births and Deaths) Regs 1982 (SI 1982 No 286)
f.   *Road Traffic Accidents*
     Road Traffic Act 1972, Sections 7–10, 154 and 155

g. *Detained Psychiatric Patients*
   Mental Health Act 1983, Sections 37 and 41
h. *Sexually Transmitted Diseases*
   The National Health Service (Venereal Diseases) Regs 1974 (SI 1974 No 29)

Annex B: Examples of Agencies with Statutory Powers to Order Disclosure

a. *The Health Service Commissioner*
   NHS Act 1977, Schedule 13
b. *Inquiry appointed by Secretary of State for Social Services*
   NHS Act 1977, Section 84
   Children Act 1975, Section 98
c. *Health and Safety Commission*
   Health and Safety Executive
   Health and Safety at Work Etc Act 1974, Section 27
d. *Employment Medical Advisers*
   Health and Safety at Work Etc Act 1974, Section 60(1)
e. *Mental Health Act Commission*
   Mental Health Act 1983, Sections 60, 120, 121

Annex C: Examples of Courts, Persons or Bodies Empowered by or Under Statute to Order Disclosure

a. *A Court of Law, including Coroners' Courts*
   The Supreme Court Act 1981
   The Rules of the Supreme Court – Order 24
   The Criminal Procedure (Attendance of Witnesses) Act 1965
   The Coroners Acts 1887–1980
b. *Mental Health Review Tribunals*
   Mental Health Act 1983. Section 78
c. *Committee or Tribunal*
   NHS (Service Committees and Tribunal) Regulations 1974 (SI 1974 No 455)

Annex D: Examples of Essential Management Functions

a. *Investigating a Complaint or Untoward Incident*
   DHSS Circulars –
   HM(55)66 – Reporting of accidents in hospitals
   HM(66)15 – Methods of dealing with complaints by patients
   Dear Secretary Letters 9/12/66 and 27/7/70
   HM(72)37 – Surgical accidents
   HC(81)5 – Health Service Complaints Procedure
b. *Responding to a Claim for Compensation and Notice of Proceedings*
   DHSS Circulars –

HM(54)32 – Legal proceedings
HM(54)43 – Legal proceedings – hospital dental staff
HM(59)88 – Supply of information to patients engaged in legal
proceedings
HM(61)110 – Supply of information about psychiatric patients
engaged in legal proceedings
HC(82)16 – Supply of information about hospital patients in the
context of civil legal proceedings

c.   *Investigating an Allegation Against a Member of Staff Concerning Patient
Care and Treatment*
DHSS Circulars – as for a. above plus:
HM(61)37 – Reports to statutory professional bodies about hospital
staff dismissals or resignations where these have been
court convictions
HM(61)112 – Disciplinary proceedings in cases relating to hospital
medical and dental staff
General Whitley Council Handbook

d.   *Exercising Powers of Discharge of Psychiatric Patients*
Mental Health Act 1983, Section 23

e.   *Mental Health Act Commission*
Mental Health Act 1983, Section 60, 120 and 121

f.   *Mental Health Review Tribunals*
Mental Health act 1983, Section 78

g.   *Local Authority Registers of Disabled Persons*
Chronically Sick and Disabled Persons Act, Section 1

h.   *Employment Registers (Manpower Services Commission)*
Disabled Persons (Employment) Act 1944

International Code of Medical Ethics
(World Medical Association, 1949, 1968, 1983)

Duties of Physicians in General

A PHYSICIAN SHALL always maintain the highest standards of professional conduct.

A PHYSICIAN SHALL not permit motives of profit to influence the free and independent exercise of professional judgment on behalf of patients.

A PHYSICIAN SHALL, in all types of medical practice, be dedicated to providing competent medical service in full technical and moral independence, with compassion and respect for human dignity.

A PHYSICIAN SHALL deal honestly with patients and colleagues, and strive to expose those physicians deficient in character or competence, or who engage in fraud or deception.

The following practices are deemed to be unethical conduct:
a) Self advertising by physicians, unless permitted by the laws of the country and the Code of Ethics of the National Medical Association.
b) Paying or receiving any fee or any other consideration solely to procure the referral of a patient or for prescribing or referring a patient to any source.

A PHYSICIAN SHALL respect the rights of patients, of colleagues, and of other health professionals, and shall safeguard patient confidences.

A PHYSICIAN SHALL act only in the patient's interest when providing medical care which might have the effect of weakening the physical and mental condition of the patient.

A PHYSICIAN SHALL use great caution in divulging discoveries or new techniques or treatment through non-professional channels.

A PHYSICIAN SHALL certify only that which he has personally verified.

Duties of Physicians to the Sick

A PHYSICIAN SHALL always bear in mind the obligation of preserving human life.

A PHYSICIAN SHALL owe his patients complete loyalty and all the resources of his science. Whenever an examination or treatment is beyond the physician's capacity he should summon another physician who has the necessary ability.

A PHYSICIAN SHALL preserve absolute confidentiality on all he knows about his patient even after the patient has died.

A PHYSICIAN SHALL give emergency care as a humanitarian duty unless he is assured that others are willing and able to give such care.

Duties of Physicians to each other

A PHYSICIAN SHALL behave towards his colleagues as he would have them behave towards him.

A PHYSICIAN SHALL NOT entice patients from his colleagues.

A PHYSICIAN SHALL observe the principles of the "Declaration of Geneva" approved by the World Medical Association.

Regulations in Time of Armed Conflict (World Medical Association, 1956, 1957, 1983)

1. Medical Ethics in time of armed conflict is identical to medical ethics in time of peace, as established in the International Code of Medical Ethics of the World Medical Association. The primary obligation of the physician is his professional duty; in performing his professional duty, the physician's supreme guide is his conscience.

2. The primary task of the medical profession is to preserve health and save life. Hence it is deemed unethical for physicians to:
   A. Give advice or perform prophylactic, diagnostic or therapeutic procedures that are not justifiable in the patient's interest.
   B Weaken the physical or mental strength of a human being without therapeutic justification.
   C Employ scientific knowledge or imperil health or destroy life.

3. Human experimentation in time of armed conflict is governed by the same code as in time of peace; it is strictly forbidden on all persons deprived of their liberty, especially civilian and military prisoners and the population of occupied countries.

4. In emergencies, the physician must always give the

required care impartially and without consideration of sex, race, nationality, religion, political affiliation or any other similar criterion. Such medical assistance must be continued for as long as necessary and practicable.

5. Medical confidentiality must be preserved by the physician in the practice of his profession.

6. Privileges and facilities afforded the physician must never be used for other than professional purposes.

Rules governing the care of sick and wounded, particularly in time of conflict

A. 1. Under all circumstances, every person, military or civilian must receive promptly the care he needs without consideration of sex, race, nationality, religion, political affiliation or any other similar criterion.

2. Any procedure detrimental to the health, physical or mental integrity of a human being is forbidden unless therapeutically justifiable.

B. 1. In emergencies, physicians and associated medical personnel are required to render immediate service to the best of their ability. No distinction shall be made between patients except those justified by medical urgency.

2. The members of medical and auxiliary professions must be granted the protection needed· to carry out their professional activities freely. The assistance necessary should be given to them in fulfilling their responsibilities. Free passage should be granted whenever their assistance is required. They should be afforded complete professional independence.

3. The fulfillment of medical duties and responsibilities shall in no circumstances be considered an offence.

The physician must never be prosecuted for observing professional secrecy.

4. In fulfilling their professional duties, the medical and auxiliary professions will be identified by the distinctive emblem of a red serpent and staff on a white field. The use of this emblem is governed by special regulation.

Resolution on Physician Participation in Capital Punishment
(World Medical Association, 1981)

Following concern about the introduction of an execution method (lethal injection) which threatened to involve doctors directly in the process of execution, the WMA Secretary-General issued a press statement opposing any involvement of doctors in capital punishment. The 34th Assembly of the WMA, meeting in Lisbon some weeks after the issuing of the press statement, endorsed the Secretary-General's statement in the following terms:

Resolution on Physician Participation in Capital Punishment

RESOLVED, that the Assembly of the World Medical Association endorses the action of the Secretary General in issuing the attached press release on behalf of the World Medical Association condemning physician participation in capital punishment.

FURTHER RESOLVED, that it is unethical for physicians to participate in capital punishment, although this does not preclude physicians certifying death.

FURTHER RESOLVED, that the Medical Ethics Committee keep this matter under active consideration.

Secretary General's Press Release

The first capital punishment by intravenous injection of

lethal dose of drugs was decided to be carried out next week by the court of the State of Oklahoma, USA.

Regardless of the method of capital punishment a State imposes, no physician should be required to be an active participant. Physicians are dedicated to preserving life.

Acting as an executioner is not the practice of medicine and physician services are not required to carry out capital punishment even if the methodology utilizes pharmacological agents or equipment that might otherwise be used in the practice of medicine.

A physician's only role would be to certify death once the State had carried out the capital punishment.

September 11, 1981

The Declaration of Geneva
(World Medical Association, 1948, 1968, 1983)

AT THE TIME OF BEING ADMITTED AS A MEMBER OF THE MEDICAL PROFESSION:

I SOLEMNLY PLEDGE myself to consecrate my life to the service of humanity;

I WILL GIVE to my teachers the respect and gratitude which is their due;

I WILL PRACTICE my profession with conscience and dignity;

THE HEALTH OF MY PATIENT will be my first consideration;

I WILL RESPECT the secrets which are confided in me, even after the patient has died;

I WILL MAINTAIN by all means in my power, the honor and the noble traditions of the medical profession;

MY COLLEAGUES will be my brothers;

I WILL NOT PERMIT considerations of religion, nationality, race, party politics or social standing to intervene between my duty and my patient;

I WILL MAINTAIN the utmost respect for human life from its beginning even under threat and I will not use my medical knowledge contrary to the laws of humanity;

I MAKE THESE PROMISES solemnly, freely and upon my honor.

The Declaration of Helsinki
(World Medical Association, 1964, 1975)

Introduction
It is the mission of the medical doctor to safeguard the health of the people. His or her knowledge and conscience are dedicated to the fulfilment of this mission.

The Declaration of Geneva of the World Medical Association binds the doctor with the words, "The health of my patient will be my first consideration," and the International Code of Medical Ethics declares that, "Any act or advice which could weaken physical or mental resistance of a human being may be used only in his interest."

The purpose of biomedical research involving human subjects must be to improve diagnostic, therapeutic and prophylactic procedures and the understanding of the aetiology and pathogenesis of disease.

In current medical practice most diagnostic, therapeutic or prophylactic procedures involve hazards. This applies *a fortiori* to biomedical research.

Medical progress is based on research which ultimately must rest in part on experimentation involving human subjects.

In the field of biomedical research a fundamental distinction must be recognised between medical research in which the aim is essentially diagnostic or therapeutic for a patient, and medical research, the essential object of which is purely scientific and without direct diagnostic or therapeutic value to the person subjected to the research.

Special caution must be exercised in the conduct of research which may affect the environment, and the welfare of animals used for research must be respected.

Because it is essential that the results of laboratory experiments be applied to human beings to further scientific knowledge and to help suffering humanity, The World Medical Association has prepared the following recommendations as a guide to every doctor in biomedical research involving human subjects. They should be kept under review in the future. It must be stressed that the standards as drafted are only a guide to physicians all over the world. Doctors are not relieved from criminal, civil and ethical responsibilities under the laws of their own countries.

I. Basic principles

1. Biomedical research involving human subjects must conform to generally accepted scientific principles and should be based on adequately performed laboratory and animal experimentation and on a thorough knowledge of the scientific literature.

2. The design and performance of each experimental procedure involving human subjects should be clearly formulated in an experimental protocol which should be transmitted to a specially appointed independent committee for consideration, comment and guidance.

3. Biomedical research involving human subjects should be conducted only by scientifically qualified persons and under the supervision of a clinically competent medical person. The responsibility for the human subject must always rest with a medically qualified person and never rest on the subject of the research, even though the subject has given his or her consent.

4. Biomedical research involving human subjects cannot legitimately be carried out unless the importance of the objective is in proportion to the inherent risk to the subject.

5. Every biomedical research project involving human subjects should be preceded by careful assessment of predictable risks in comparison with foreseeable benefits to the subject or to others. Concern for the interests of the subject

must always prevail over the interests of science and society.

6. The right of the research subject to safeguard his or her integrity must always be respected. Every precaution should be taken to respect the privacy of the subject and to minimize the impact of the study on the subject's physical and mental integrity and on the personality of the subject.

7. Doctors should abstain from engaging in research projects involving human subjects unless they are satisfied that the hazards involved are believed to be predictable. Doctors should cease any investigation if the hazards are found to outweigh the potential benefits.

8. In the publication of the results of his or her research, the doctor is obliged to preserve the accuracy of the results. Reports of experimentation not in accordance with the principles laid down in this Declaration should not be accepted for publication.

9. In any research on human beings, each potential subject must be adequately informed of the aims, methods, anticipated benefits and potential hazards of the study and the discomfort it may entail. He or she should be informed that he or she is at liberty to abstain from participation in the study and that he or she is free to withdraw his or her consent to participation at any time. The doctor should then obtain the subject's freely-given informed consent, preferably in writing.

10. When obtaining informed consent for the research project the doctor should be particularly cautious if the subject is in a dependent relationship to him or her or may consent under duress. In that case the informed consent should be obtained by a doctor who is not engaged in the investigation and who is completely independent of this official relationship.

11. In case of legal incompetence, informed consent should be obtained from the legal guardian in accordance with

national legislation. Where physical or mental incapacity makes it impossible to obtain informed consent or when the subject is a minor, permission from the responsible relative replaces that of the subject in accordance with national legislation.

12. The research protocol should always contain a statement of the ethical considerations involved and should indicate that the principles enunciated in the present Declaration are complied with.

II. Medical research combined with professional care
(Clinical research)

1. In the treatment of a sick person, the doctor must be free to use a new diagnostic and therapeutic measure, if in his or her judgment it offers hope of saving life, re-establishing health or alleviating suffering.

2. The potential benefits, hazards and discomfort of a new method should be weighed against the advantages of the best current diagnostic and therapeutic methods.

3. In any medical study, every patient—including those of a control group, if any—should be assured of the best proven diagnostic and therapeutic method.

4. The refusal of the patient to participate in a study must never interfere with the doctor–patient relationship.

5. If the doctor considers it essential not to obtain informed consent, the specific reasons for this proposal should be stated in the experimental protocol for transmission to the independent committee.

6. The doctor can combine medical research with professional care, the objective being the acquisition of new medical knowledge, only to the extent that medical research is justified by its potential diagnostic or therapeutic value for the patient.

III. Non-therapeutic biomedical research involving human subjects (Non-clinical biomedical research)

1. In the purely scientific application of medical research carried out on a human being, it is the duty of the doctor to remain the protector of the life and health of that person on whom biomedical research is being carried out.

2. The subjects should be volunteers—either healthy persons or patient for whom the experimental design is not related to the patient's illness.

3. The investigator or the investigating team should discontinue the research if in his/her or their judgment it may, if continued, be harmful to the individual.

4. In research on man, the interest of science and society should never take precedence over considerations related to the well-being of the subject.

The Declaration of Oslo (World Medical Association, 1970)

In 1970 the World Medical Association drew up a Statement on Therapeutic Abortion. This code, known as the Declaration of Oslo, was amended by the 35th World Medical Assembly, Venice, Italy, in October 1983, and states:

(1) The first moral principle imposed upon the physician is respect for human life from its beginning.
(2) Circumstances which bring the vital interests of a mother into conflict with the vital interests of her unborn child create a dilemma and raise the question whether or not the pregnancy should be deliberately terminated.
(3) Diversity of response to this situation results from the diversity of attitudes towards the life of the unborn child. This is a matter of individual conviction and conscience which must be respected.
(4) It is not the role of the medical profession to

determine the attitudes and rules of any particular state or community in this matter, but it is our duty to attempt both to ensure the protection of our patients and to safeguard the rights of the physician within society.

(5) Therefore, where the law allows therapeutic abortion to be performed, the procedure should be performed by a physician competent to do so in premises approved by the appropriate authority.

(6) If the physician considers that his convictions do not allow him to advise or perform an abortion, he may withdraw while ensuring the continuity of (medical) care by a qualified colleague.

(7) This statement, while it is endorsed by the General Assembly of the World Medical Association, is not to be regarded as binding on any individual member association unless it is adopted by that member association.

The Declaration of Sydney
(World Medical Association, 1968)

The World Medical Association formulated a Statement on Death in 1968. Known as the Declaration of Sydney, it was amended by the 35th World Medical Assembly in Venice, Italy, in 1983, and reads:

(1) The determination of the time of death is in most countries the legal responsibility of the physician and should remain so. Usually the physician will be able without special assistance to decide that a person is dead, employing the classical criteria known to all physicians.

(2) Two modern practices in medicine, however, have made it necessary to study the question of the time of death further: (a) the ability to maintain by artificial means the circulation of oxygenated blood through tissues of the body which may have been irreversibly injured and (b) the use of cadaver organs such as heart or kidneys for transplantation.

(3) A complication is that death is a gradual process at the cellular level with tissues varying in their ability to

withstand deprivation of oxygen. But clinical interest lies
not in the state of preservation of isolated cells but in the
fate of a person. Here the point of death of the different
cells and organs is not so important as the certainty that
the process has become irreversible by whatever techniques of resuscitation that may be employed.

(4) It is essential to determine the irreversible cessation of
all functions of the entire brain, including the brain stem.
This determination will be based on clinical judgment
supplemented if necessary by a number of diagnostic
aids. However, no single technological criterion is
entirely satisfactory in the present state of medicine nor
can any one technological procedure be substituted for
the overall judgment of the physician. If transplantation
of an organ is involved, the decision that death exists
should be made by two or more physicians and the
physicians determining the moment of death should in
no way be immediately concerned with the performance
of the transplantation.

(5) Determination of the point of death of the person
makes it ethically permissible to cease attempts at
resuscitation and in countries where the law permits, to
remove organs from the cadaver provided that prevailing
legal requirements of consent have been fulfilled.

The Declaration of Tokyo
(World Medical Association, 1975)

It is the privilege of the medical doctor to practise medicine in
the service of humanity, to preserve and restore bodily and
mental health without distinction as to persons, to comfort
and to ease the suffering of his or her patients. The utmost
respect for human life is to be maintained even under threat,
and no use made of any medical knowledge contrary to the
laws of humanity.

For the purpose of this Declaration, torture is defined as
the deliberate, systematic or wanton infliction of physical or
mental suffering by one or more persons acting alone or on

the orders of any authority, to force another person to yield information, to make a confession, or for any other reason.

1. The doctor shall not countenance, condone or participate in the practice of torture or other forms of cruel, inhuman or degrading procedures, whatever the offence of which the victim of such procedures is suspected, accused or guilty, and whatever the victim's beliefs or motives, and in all situations, including armed conflict and civil strife.

2. The doctor shall not provide any premises, instruments, substances or knowledge to facilitate the practice of torture or other forms of cruel, inhuman or degrading treatment or to diminish the ability of the victim to resist such treatment.

3. The doctor shall not be present during any procedure during which torture or other forms of cruel, inhuman or degrading treatment is used or threatened.

4. A doctor must have complete clinical independence in deciding upon the care of a person for whom he or she is medically responsible. The doctor's fundamental role is to alleviate the distress of his or her fellow men, and no motive whether personal, collective or political shall prevail against this higher purpose.

5. Where a prisoner refuses nourishment and is considered by the doctor as capable of forming an unimpaired and rational judgment concerning the consequences of such a voluntary refusal of nourishment, he or she shall not be fed artificially. The decision as to the capacity of the prisoner to form such a judgment should be confirmed by at least one other independent doctor. The consequences of the refusal of nourishment shall be explained by the doctor to the prisoner.

6. The World Medical Association will support, and should encourage the international community, the national

medical associations and fellow doctors, to support the doctor and his or her family in the face of threats or reprisals resulting from a refusal to condone the use of torture or other forms of cruel, inhuman or degrading treatment.

SELECT BIBLIOGRAPHY

Main sources

Beauchamp, Tom L. and Childress, James F., *Principles of Biomedical Ethics*, Oxford University Press, New York 1979.

Bloch, Sidney and Chodoff, Paul, *Psychiatric Ethics*, Oxford University Press, 1981.

British Medical Association, *Medical Ethics 1970*.
 The Handbook of Medical Ethics 1983.

Campbell, A.V., *Moral Dilemmas in Medicine*, Churchill Livingstone 1975.

Glover, Jonathan, *Causing Death and Saving Lives*, Penguin 1977.

Kennedy, Ian, *The Unmasking of Medicine*, Paladin 1983.

Mason and McCall Smith, *Law and Medical Ethics*, Butterworths 1983.

McLean, Sheila and Maher, Gerry, *Medicine, Morals and the Law*, Gower 1983.

Mill, J.S., *On Liberty*, Penguin 1982.

Pellegrino, E. and Thomasma, D., *A Philosophical Basis of Medical Practice*, Oxford University Press 1981.

Veatch, Robert M., *A Theory of Medical Ethics*, Basic Books Inc. New York 1981.

Additional references

Lorber, J, 'Selective treatment of myelomeningocele', *Paediatrics*, vol. 53, no. 3. March 1974.
 'Ethical problems in the management of myelomeningocele and hydrocephalus', *Journal of the Royal College of Physicians*, vol. 10, no. 1, 1975.

Council for Science and Society, *Life and Death Before Birth*, 1978.

Department of Health and Social Security, 'Priorities for health and personal social services in England', a consultative document, HMSO 1976.
 'Inequalities in health: report of a research working group', 1980.

Mitchell, Basil, 'Is a moral consensus in medical ethics possible?' *Journal of Medical Ethics*, 2, 18 March 1976.

President's Commission for the Study of Ethical Problems in Medicine and Biomedical and Behavioural Research, *Securing*

Access to Health Care, March 1983.

Plant, Raymond, 'The greatest happiness', *Journal of Medical Ethics*, 1, July 1975.

Hare, Richard, 'Medical ethics: can the moral philosopher help?' 1977 (in *Philosophical Medical Ethics: Its Nature and Significance*, ed. Spicker, S.F. and Engelhardt Jnr, H.T.

Harris, John, 'Ethical problems in the management of some severely handicapped children', *Journal of Medical Ethics*, 7, 1981.

'Withholding treatment in infancy', *British Medical Journal*, 21 March 1981.

'Thou shalt not strive officiously', *British Medical Journal*, 13 November 1982.

'Death without concealment', *British Medical Journal*, 19–26 December 1981.

'The right to live and the right to die', *British Medical Journal*, 29 August 1981.

Brahams, Diana and Malcolm: 'The Arthur case: a proposal for legislation', *Journal of Medical Ethics*, 9, March 1983.

Campbell, A.G.M. and Duff, R.S., 'Deciding the care of severely malformed or dying infants', *Journal of Medical Ethics*, 5, 1979.

Acheson, Roy M, 'The definition and identification of need for health care'. *Journal of Epidemiology and Community Health*, 32, 1978.

'Paediatricians and the law', *British Medical Journal*, 14 November 1981.

Havard, J, 'Legislation is likely to create more difficulty than it resolves', *Journal of Medical Ethics*, 9, 1983.

Campbell, A.G.M. 'Which infants should not receive intensive care?' Archives of Disease in Childhood, 57, 1982.

'After the trial at Leicester', *The Lancet*, 14 November 1981.

Kottow, Michael, 'Medical ethics: who decides what?' *Journal of Medical Ethics*, 9, 1983.

'The doctor as inquisitor', *The Lancet*, 1 April 1972.

'The doctor in conflict', *British Medical Journal*, 25 March 1972.

'Who shall die?' *Journal of Medical Ethics*, 6, 1980.

'What price life?' *The Lancet*, 9 October 1982.

Tudor Hart, Julian, 'A lottery for life', letter to *The Lancet*, 20 Augustm 1983.

Abel-Smith, Brian, 'Health care in a cold economic climate', *The Lancet*, 14 February 1981.

Knox, E.G. 'Principles of allocation of health care resources', *Journal of Epidemiology and Community Health*, 32, 1978.

'What a RAWProar', *British Medical Journal*, 27 November 1976.

Campbell, A.V., 'Establishing ethical priorities in medicine', *British Medical Journal*, 26 March 1977.

Parsons, V. and Lock, P., 'Triage and the patient with renal failure', *Journal of Medical Ethics*, 6, 1980.

Sagan, Leonard and Jonsen, Albert, 'Medical ethics and torture', *New England Journal of Medicine*, 294, 1976.

'The Declaration of Tokyo: no truck with torture', *The Medical Journal of Australia*, 15 November 1975.

Jones, Gray E, 'On the permissibility of torture', *Journal of Medical Ethics*, 6, 1980.

Kennedy, Ian, 'The Karen Quinlan case; problems and proposals', *Journal of Medical Ethics*, 2, 1976.

'Genetic counselling and the prevention of Huntington's Chorea', *The Lancet*, 16 January 1982.

'Research on embryos: ethics under fire', *New Scientist*, 30 September 1982.

Grobstein, Clifford, 'Coming to terms with test-tube babies', *New Scientist*, 7 October 1982.

Edwards, R.G., 'Test-tube babies: the ethical debate', *The Listener*, 27 October 1983.

'Research on infants', *The Lancet*, 14 May 1977.

Beedie, Margaret A., and Bluglass, Robert; 'Consent to psychiatric treatment: practical considerations of the Mental Health (Amendment) Bill', *British Medical Journal*, 29 May 1982.

Gostin, Larry O, 'Psychosurgery: a hazardous and unestablished treatment?' *Journal of Social Welfare Law*, 1982.

'Controlled trials: planned deception?' *The Lancet*, 10 March 1979.

'Randomised controlled trials?' *British Medical Journal*, 17 November 1979.

Cancer Research Campaign Working Party in Breast Conservation, 'Informed consent: ethical, legal and medical implications for doctors and patients who participate in randomised clinical trials', *British Medical Journal*, 2 April 1983.

Brewin, Thurstan B, 'Consent to randomised treatment?' *The Lancet*, 23 October 1982.

Vere, D.W., 'Problems in controlled trials: a critical response', *Journal of Medical Ethics*, 9, 1983.

Burkhardt, R. and Kienle, G., 'Basic problems in controlled trials', *Journal of Medical Ethics*, 9, 1983.

Kirby, Michael, 'Informed consent: what does it mean?' *Journal of Medical Ethics*, 9, 1983.

'Secret randomised clinical trials', *The Lancet*, 10 July 1983.

Lyndon Wade, Owen, 'Informed consent to clinical trials in cancer', letter to The Lancet, 31 July 1982.

Thomas, S. 'Ethics of a predictive test for Huntington's Chorea', *British Medical Journal*, 8 May 1982.

Arnold, A. and Moseley, R. 'Ethical issues arising from human genetics', *Journal of Medical Ethics*, 2, 1976.

Seller, Mary J, 'Ethical aspects of genetic counselling', *Journal of Medical Ethics*, 8, 1982.
Royal College of Obstetricians and Gynaecologists, 'Report of the RCOG ethics committee on IVF and embryo replacement or transfer', 1983.
Royal College of General Practitioners, 'Evidence to the government inquiry into human fertilisation and embryology', 1983.
Kincaid-Smith, Priscilla, 'Ethics and IVF', *British Medical Journal*, 1 May 1982.
Kirby, Michael, *IVF: the Scope and Limitation of Law*, 1983.
Godber, George, 'Striking the balance; therapy, prevention and support', *World Health Forum*, 3, 1982.
Institute of Society Ethics and the Life Sciences; *Biomedical Ethics and the Shadow of Nazism*, 1976.
Burges, Stanley H., 'Doctors and torture: the police surgeon', *Journal of Medical Ethics*, 6, 1980.
Bowden, Paul, 'Medical practice: defendants and prisoners', *Journal of Medical Ethics*, 2, 1976.
'Report of the inquiry into allegations against the security forces of physical brutality in Northern Ireland arising out of events on 9 August 1971', HMSO, 1971.
Prewer, R, 'The contribution of prison medicine', (in *Progress in Penal Reform*; ed. Blom-Cooper, L., Clarendon Press 1974).
British Medical Association, *The Occupational Physician*, 1980.
'Professional secrecy', *British Medical Journal*, 28 May 1966.
Hodges, Catherine, 'When the police come knocking at your door', *Pulse*, 14 June 1980.
Hall, Anthony, 'Illegal immigration and medical confidentiality', letter to *British Medical Journal*, 23 February 1980.
Phillips, Melanie, 'Ministry tells doctors to spy on migrants', *Guardian*, 5 December 1979
   'Virginity tests on immigrants at Heathrow', *Guardian*, 1 February 1979.
'Asian emigrants X-rayed by UK officials', *Guardian*, 8 February 1979.
Kenny, D.J., 'Confidentiality: the confusion continues', *Journal of Medical Ethics*, 8, 1982.
Thompson, Ian E., 'The nature of confidentiality', *Journal of Medical Ethics*, 5, 1979.
Galbraith, S., 'The "no lose" philosophy in medicine', *Journal of Medical Ethics*, 4, 1978.

INDEX